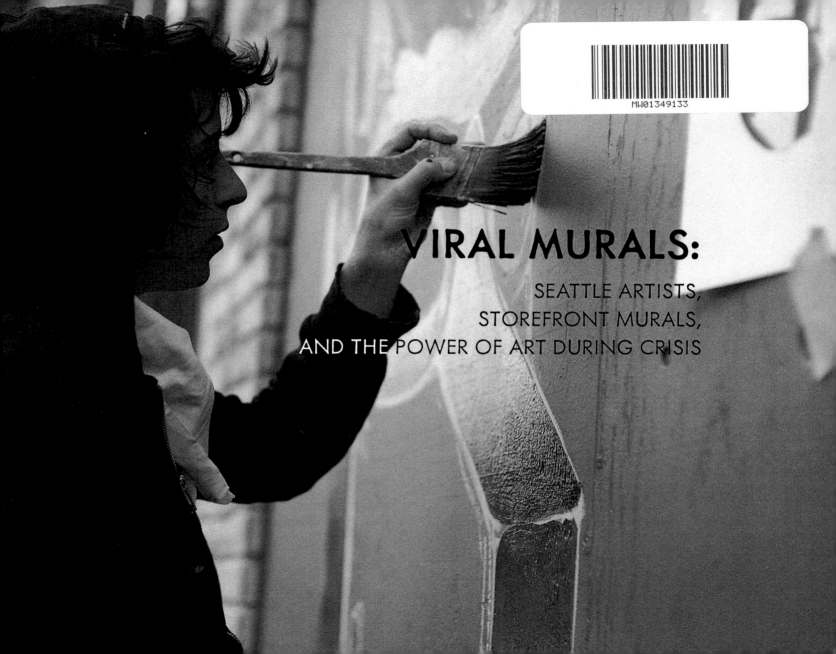

VIRAL MURALS:

SEATTLE ARTISTS,
STOREFRONT MURALS,
AND THE POWER OF ART DURING CRISIS

THIS IS TEMPORARY

VIRAL MURALS:

SEATTLE ARTISTS,
STOREFRONT MURALS,
AND THE POWER OF ART DURING CRISIS

Conceived and edited by Annie Brulé & Phil Bevis
With the assistance of Dean Kelly, Malia Maxwell, & Cyra Jane Hobson

CHATWIN BOOKS
2020

Viral Murals: Seattle Artists, Storefront Murals, and the Power of Art During Crisis, copyright Chatwin LLC, 2020.

All artwork copyright the respective artists; all photographs copyright the respective photographers; all text and quotes copyright the respective authors. All editorial, curation, arrangement, and book design copyright Chatwin Books.

No part of this book may be reproduced via means either print, digital, electronic or otherwise, without written permission of the publisher, except for brief excerpts used in articles and publicity.

Front cover photos, clockwise from top left: *Stay Strong* by Dozfy, photo by the artist. Katlyn Hubner with their mural, *Doghouse*, photo by Steve Gilbert. Carol Rashawnna Williams with their mural, *Love, Hope, Believe, and Care in the time of COVID-19*, photo by Jordan Somers. *A Book Is A Dream* by Amanda Joyce Bishop, photo by Ty Kreft. Crystal Barbre and Casey Weldon with their mural, *Hello?*, photo by Austin Wilson. Paul Nunn with their mural, *Wave to a Stranger*, photo by the artist. *Bowie Magic* by Ronnie Taylor, photo by Austin Wilson.
Half-title photograph: Katlyn Hubner by Steve Gilbert.
Photo opposite title page: *This is Temporary* by Lance Lobuzzetta.
Artist photos (pgs 4-5), from left: Crystal Barbre by Austin Wilson, Jillian Chong and crew by Elise Wang, Ezra Dickinson by Austin Wilson.

Cover design: Annie Brulé. Interior design: Annie Brulé & Cyra Jane Hobson.
Index by Malia Maxwell.

Artists' quotations have been edited for length and context.

ISBN: 978-1633981218

Chatwin Books
www.chatwinbooks.com

Contents

Artists' Quotes......................6

Murals by Neighborhood..........9

Acknowledgements....................210

Map of Mural Locations...................211

Donors and Sponsors...........................212

Index..213

IN SPRING 2020, AS THE COVID-19 pandemic forced hundreds of businesses to close their doors and board their windows, the role of main streets in Seattle transformed. Artists, community leaders, businesses, and funders sprang into action to create vibrant, wildly diverse, uplifting art on boarded up storefronts to inspire generosity, patience, and solidarity during difficult times. The transformation of main streets into public galleries within a few weeks reminds us how vibrant community places help to build resilience, and of the wealth of latent creativity we posses, just looking for a canvas.

—from the map by Ian Crozier and Annie Brulé (see p. 211)

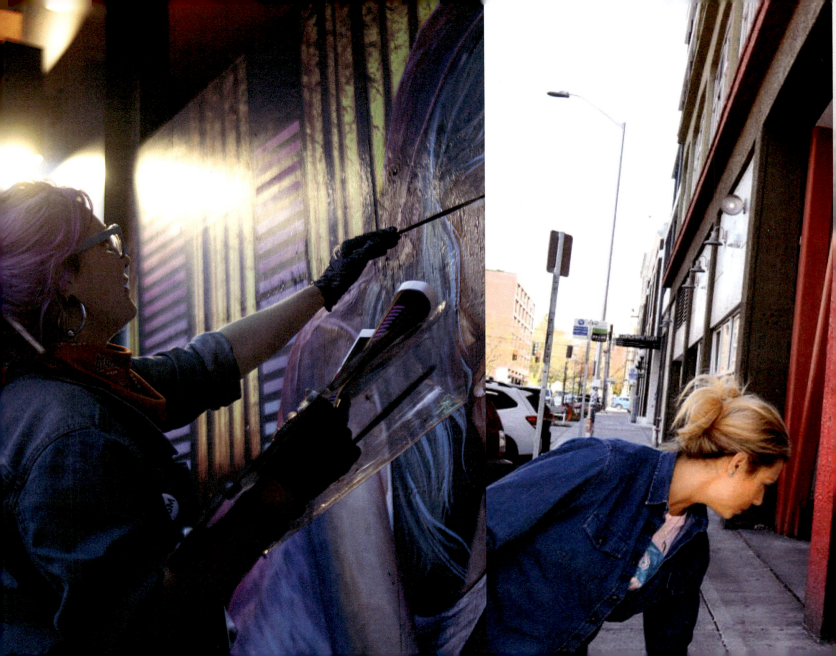

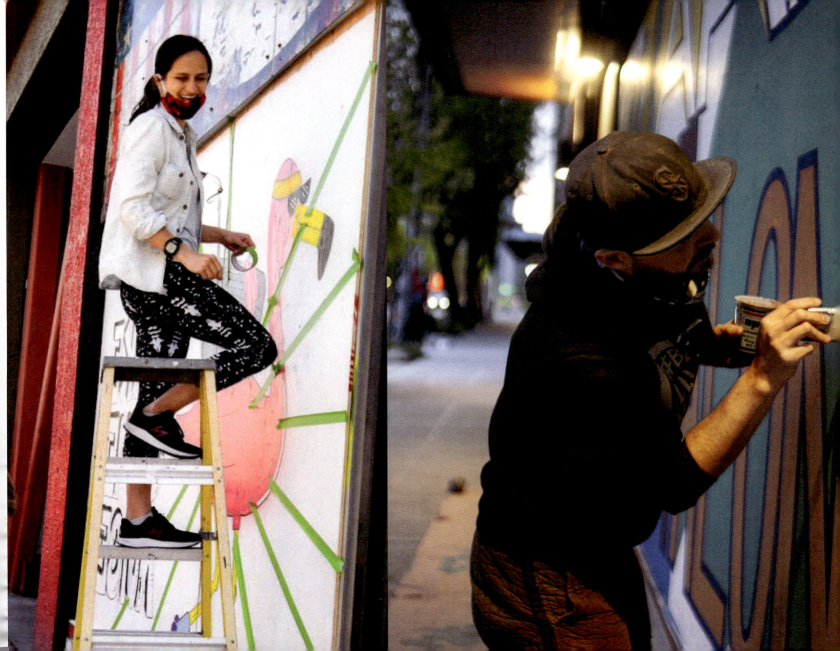

Why did you decide to do this?

Editor's note: Many of the following artists' texts have been abridged and edited for clarity and punctuation.

This was something I could contribute to to help raise morale. It also allowed me to process my emotions through art, to be surrounded by other creatives while we painted on the streets together (albeit from 6 ft away), and helped me feel more in touch with community during a time of isolation and quarantine.

—Amanda Joyce Bishop

Seemingly overnight, we transformed an eerily quiet and bleak scene into colorful streets filled with art. Rarely does an opportunity exist when artists get to come together to paint an entire neighborhood and be a part of a cohesive community message of hope.

—Lance Lobuzzetta

I painted this as a salute to women in the medical field on the front lines of the pandemic. The woman in my piece honors all of the women before her and all the women after her. She is Essential.

—Jay Mason

As a muralist in food service, I painted to reestablish my connection to a job I miss and to create a positive visual for the Pike Place Market neighborhood, which has been hit particularly hard by this crisis.

—Devon Midori Hale

I wanted to support my community during the pandemic, a crisis that further intensified the divide between the rich and poor. Street art can bring art to those who otherwise may not be able to access it. And in these circumstances, access to art has a whole new meaning, with venues and galleries closed.

—Glynn Rosenberg

I agreed to paint this mural of David Bowie on Broadway to celebrate the LGBT community. Since this is my first mural, I learned that while taking risks like this might seem scary, it's how you grow. Your soul stretches out into new horizons and abilities to be discovered. Not only in art, but also in life.

—Ronnie Taylor

I am not a healthcare worker or grocery store employee, and, as the world was shutting down around me, I struggled to see how I could contribute or help. This has given me a way to use my skills and talents to do my part for Seattle by using my artwork to bring hope and joy to my city.

—Sydney M. Pertl

Watching familiar and beloved businesses board up windows quickly transformed the street into a disparaging scene. Murals were a great way to brighten up the streetscape during this uncertain time.

—Tori Shao

When businesses first started boarding up their storefronts, Crystal and I got to talking about what a shame it was to see all of this ugly plywood and we wondered if any of them would be interested in letting us decorate them. It was the least we could do!

—Casey Weldon

I wanted to bring some positive vibes and color to the neighborhood in defiance of closed businesses and quarantine to brighten someone's day and have viewers know that this too shall pass.

—Dillon Bennet

Seattle used to have a lot more murals. However, many of those have started to disappear from our streets. On one hand, our architecture has changed—buildings are tall glass towers with little room for large pieces of art. On the other hand, the same growth that gives Seattle life has also presented many challenges for certain communities, including the artist community. Murals themselves have started to become indoor fixtures of offices rather than public pieces. Yet as I grabbed some stencils and a few cans, I saw the artist community rally behind a common goal. Because of COVID-19, that dispersed group has found a common place again: the streets. With boarded-up businesses a bittersweet opportunity was afforded that allowed us to spread a message of hope, empathy, joy, frustration, or whatever else needed to be said.

—Kreau

My hope is that this mural reminds people that we can blossom even during the darkest of times, and that we really can bloom where we are planted. Even if we are homebound and social distancing, we can still stay connected to one another and do great things.

—Mia Pizzuto

This experience sealed the deal that Seattle is home—and that creatives still exist here with something to say. I am so grateful to have been a part of this movement.

—Tara Velan

I love to make people smile. My murals are meant to transform hopeless plywood boards and drab walls into positive, inspiring, and bright murals.

—Morgan Zion

I painted this mural because I feel it is important to put positive propaganda around us. As our world slowed down with quarantine and the onset of COVID-19, there was space to begin to imagine our world anew.

—Mari Shibuya

It felt like the right time to paint something that would give people a sense of peace and calm.

—Ariel Parrow

As a queer person, I wanted to create a piece that demonstrated the unity of our intersectional LGBTQ+ community during this crisis.

—Billie Avery

Painting, for me, is a religious experience, something I feel within my being. The viewer, hopefully, will have their own interpretations, feelings, and experience.

—Eido

I hope this piece inspires folks to get creative with the ways they can show up to help their neighbors.

—Reed Olsen

I felt compelled to add a little art, color, and love to my neighborhood as we cope with the pandemic together.

—Jake Millett (Bubzini)

I wanted to share a message of hope and connectedness. To let people know that things happen and always will and that we will still be connected.

—Rainbow Tay

Art is powerful, and in these times it can act as a reminder that we are here to help each other, and that we will get through this together. Here's hoping these messages remind you to stay positive, stay safe, and above all else, call your mom.

—Sarah Robbins

Pioneer Square

Artist:	Amanda Joyce Bishop, Ty Kreft
Name of Mural:	*A Book Is A Dream*
Materials:	Latex paint, plywood
Size:	15 x 10 feet
Location:	Arundel Books, 212 1st Ave S
Coordinated by:	Overall Creative
Credits:	Neil Gaiman (text of quote)
Artist's website:	@purebonaventure on Instagram

"When we entered this global pandemic, I felt somewhat helpless, as I am not an essential worker or doctor by trade. I wasn't sure if there was anything I could do to help. When the call went out to artists to use their art and time towards addressing the depressing facades of beloved boarded-up businesses, I knew immediately that this was something I could to help raise morale. It allowed me to process my emotions through art, be surrounded by other creatives while we painted on the streets together (albeit from 6 ft away), and feel more in touch with the community during a time of isolation and quarantine."

—Amanda Joyce Bishop

Photos: ARTIST

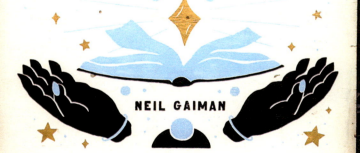
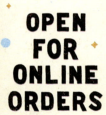
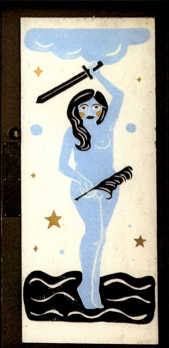

Artist: B Line Dot
Crew: Mackenzie Martin, Sam Spillman, Brandon Feely, Conor Evans
Name of Mural: *Keep Dreaming*
Materials: Spray paint, exterior house paint
Size: 12 x 18 feet
Location: Gray Sky Gallery, 320 1st Ave S.
Artist's website: blinedot.com

"My goal was to transform a boarded up doorway into something beautiful and life giving—to encourage passersby to keep dreaming, keep hoping, and keep creating."

—B Line Dot

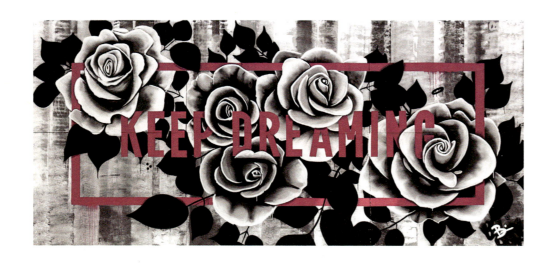

Photos: BRANDON FEELY

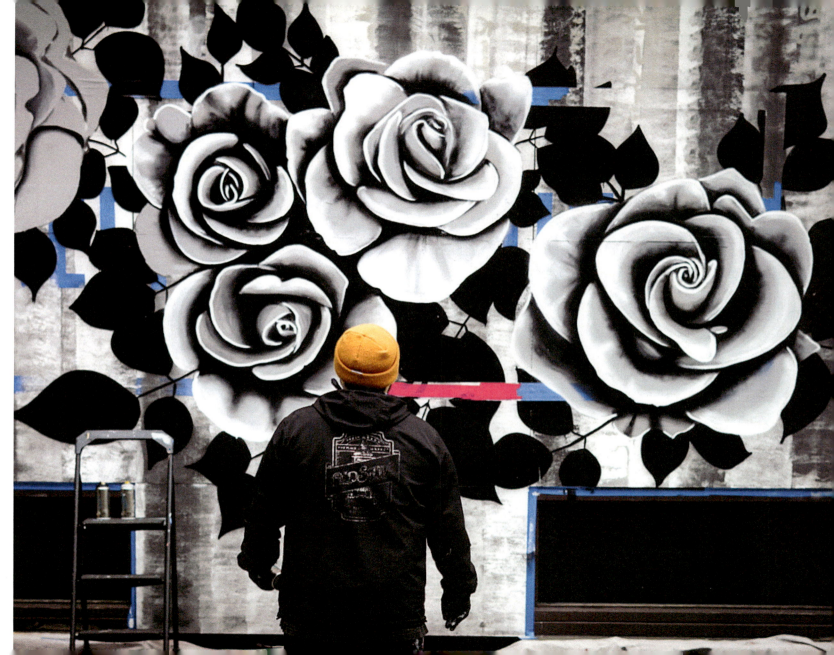

Artist:	Baso Fibonacci
Name of Mural:	*Springtime in Seattle*
Materials:	Oil enamel and acrylics
Size:	varied
Location:	Pioneer Smoke and Counter Culture Coffee, 315 1st Ave S
Coordinated by:	Pioneer Square Alliance
Artist's website:	@basofibonacci on Instagram

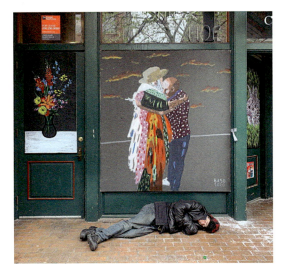 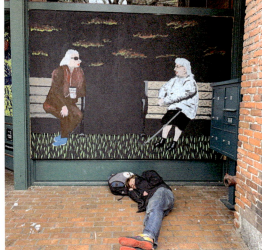

Photos: AUSTIN WILSON, ZACH ROCKSTAD

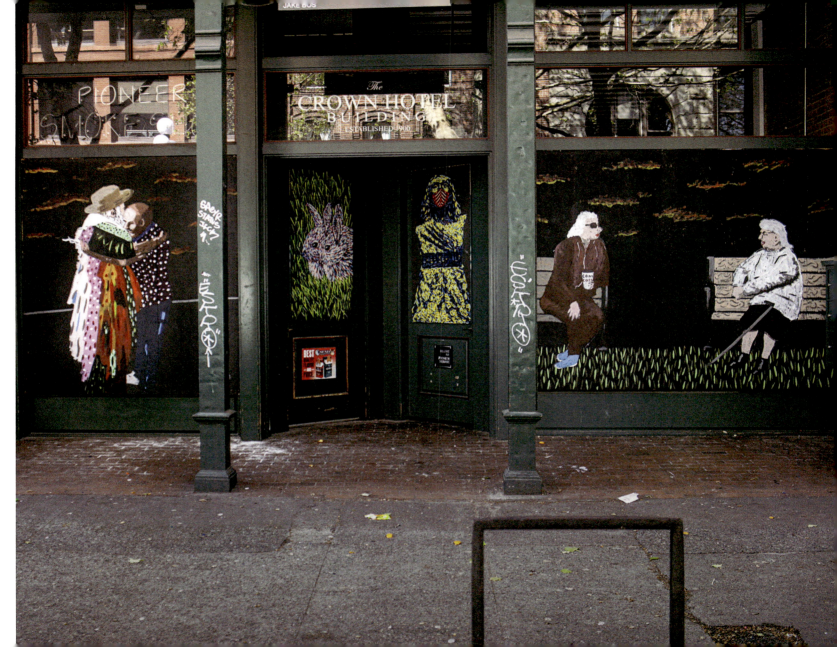

Artist: Carol Rashawnna Williams
Name of Mural: *Love, Hope, Believe, and Care in the time of COVID-19*
Materials: Outdoor paint
Size: 9 x 4 feet each
Location: Tashiro Kaplan Artists Lofts, 115 Prefontaine Pl S
Artist's website: klove4art.wixsite.com/c-rashawnna-williams

"I created the mural because I wanted to contribute to the community in a positive way."
—Carol Rashawnna Williams

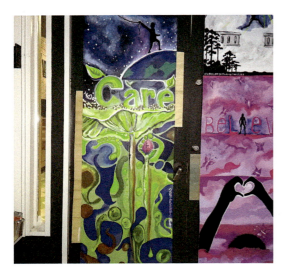
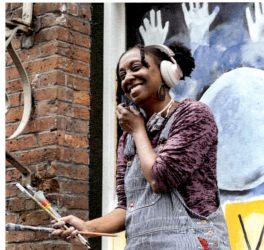
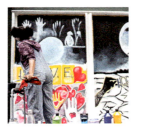

Photos: JORDAN SOMERS

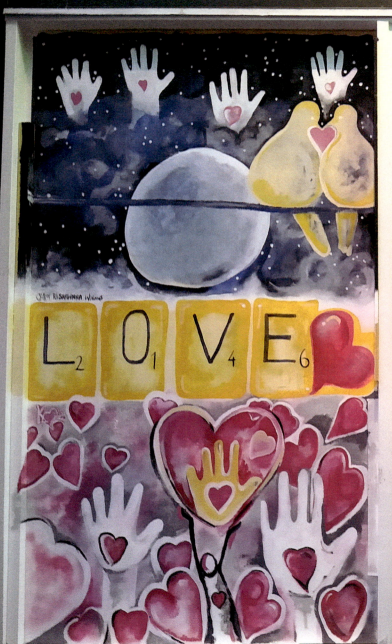
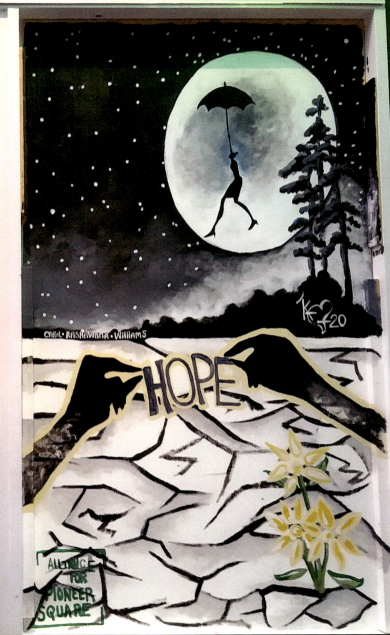

Artist: Casey Weldon
Crew: Alex Halladay, Ego
Name of Mural: *Take Your Time, Hang in There*
Materials: Acrylic paint
Size: 8 x 30 feet
Location: Bon Voyage Vintage, 110 S Washington St
Coordinated by: Alliance for Pioneer Square
Artist's website: caseyweldon.com

"I tried my best to bring something light and fun to what must be a tough time for them and other small businesses in the area."

—Casey Weldon

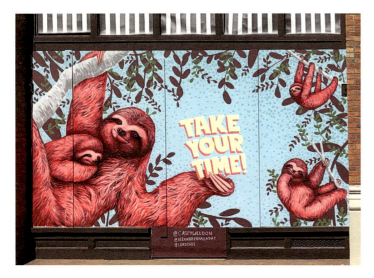
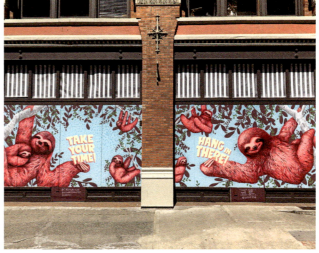

Photos: ARTIST

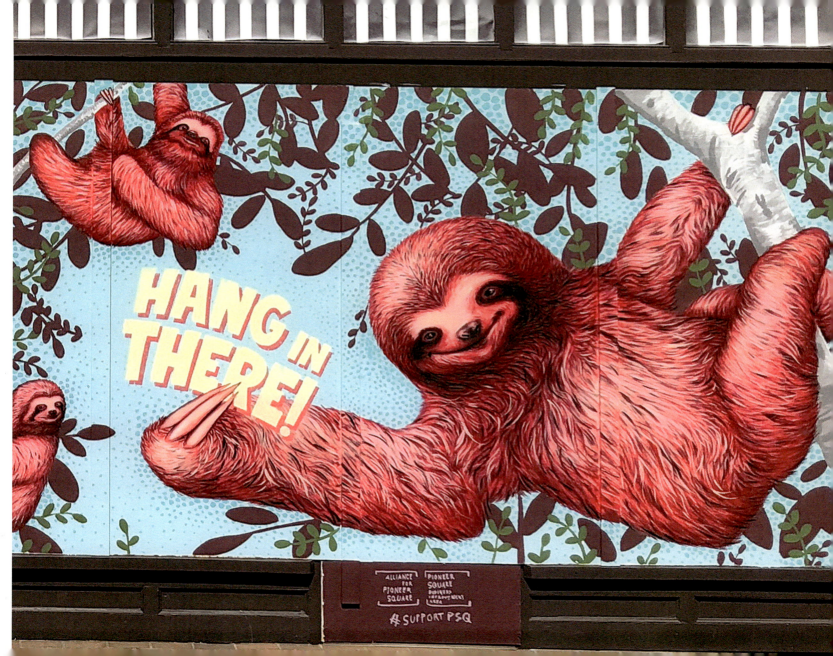

Artist: Crystal Barbre
Name of Mural: *Our Spirit Roars Courageous*
Materials: Oil paint
Size: 8 x 12 feet
Location: Gallery Erato, 309 1st Ave S
Coordinated by: Sara Pizzo
Artist's website: crystalbarbre.com

"During quarantine, people were feeling isolated and fearful of the future. Art can bring people together and contribute to an atmosphere of hope. This was what I could do to try to bring joy and beauty to the community I live in."

—Crystal Barbre

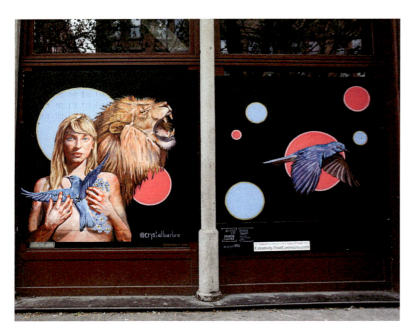
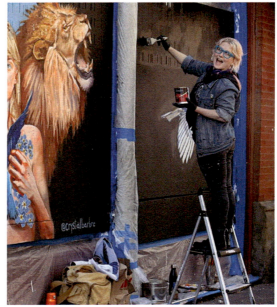

Photos: KELLY O, SCOTT MOORE

Artist:	Dawna Holloway
Crew:	Sallyann Corn, Joe Kent
Name of Mural:	*Fragrant Lemon*
Materials:	Acrylic, plywood
Size:	6 x 12 feet
Location:	fruitsuper SHOP, 524 1st Ave S
Artist's website:	studioegallery.net

"Fragrant Lemon (a group show curated by mural artist and Georgetown gallery owner Dawna Holloway of studio e gallery) was set to open April 2nd as part of First Thursday for Art Walk. This was our way of not only bringing a little joy and spot of brightness to the neighborhood, but also a way of bringing the Fragrant Lemon show from the inside to share with the outside."

—Sallyan Corn

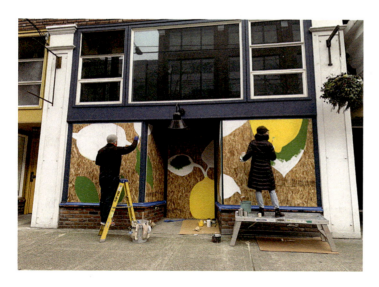
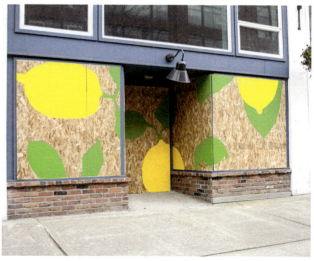

Photos: JOE KENT

Artist: Eido
Crew: Jada Love, Phineas Olafssen
Name of Mural: *The Road to Glory Stars with Love*
Materials: Acrylic paint
Size: 8 x 12 feet
Location: JuJubeet, 107 1st Ave S
Coordinated by: Sara Pizzo
Credits: Special Thanks to Tija Petrovic, Sara Pizzo
Artist's website: Poodlepublishing.com

"Painting, for me, is a religious experience, something I feel within my being. The viewer, hopefully, will have their own interpretations, feelings, and experience with the work. This is a historical event; and it is an honor to be a part of it in a positive way."

—Eido

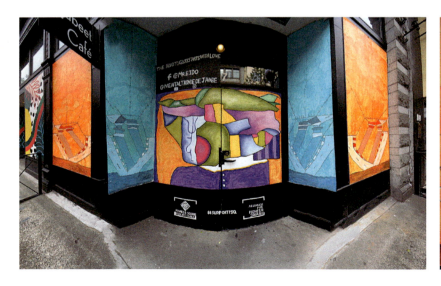 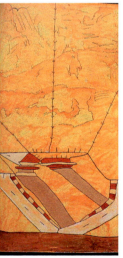 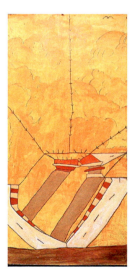

Photos: AMANDA TOLL

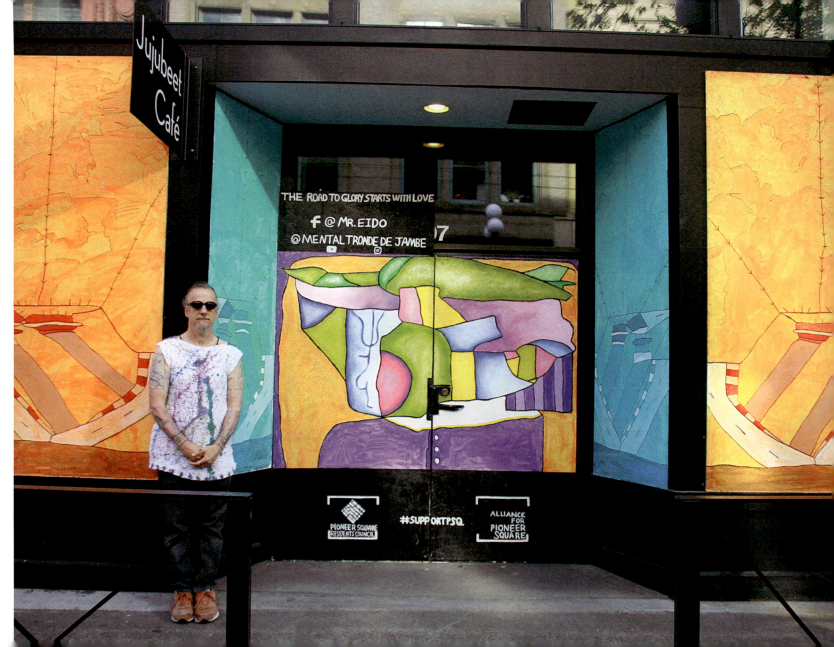

Artist:	Erin Oostra
Name of Mural:	*Remember*
Materials:	Behr paints, copper acrylic
Size:	9 x 20 feet
Location:	Kinesia Pilates Studio, 314 1st Ave S
Coordinated by:	Alliance for Pioneer Square
Credits:	Margaret Atwood (text of quote)
Artist's website:	Erinoostra.com @erinoostra on Instagram

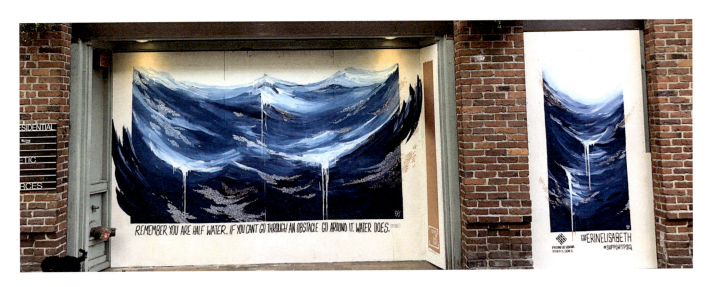

Photos: ARTIST

Artist: James the Stanton (Gnartoons)
Name of Mural: *Long Boy*
Materials: Paint
Size: varied
Location: The Grand Central Building, 216 1st Ave S
Coordinated by: Alliance for Pioneer Square
Artist's website: gnartoons.com

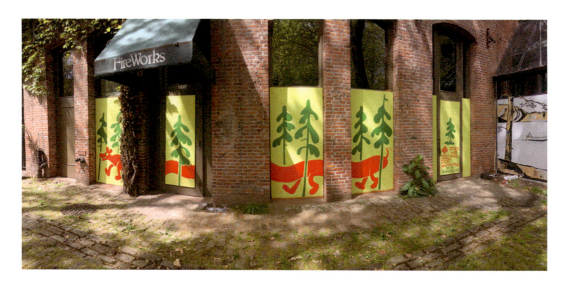

Photos: KAT WONG

Artist: Japhy Witte
Name of Mural: *Untitled*
Materials: Spray paint, latex and acrylic paint, oil enamel
Size: 8 x 11 feet each
Location: Good Bar, 240 2nd Ave S
Coordinated by: Dom Nieri
Artist's website: Signsavant.com

"I took on this project because my hands and mind needed use and my thoughts a point of expression."

—Japhy Witte

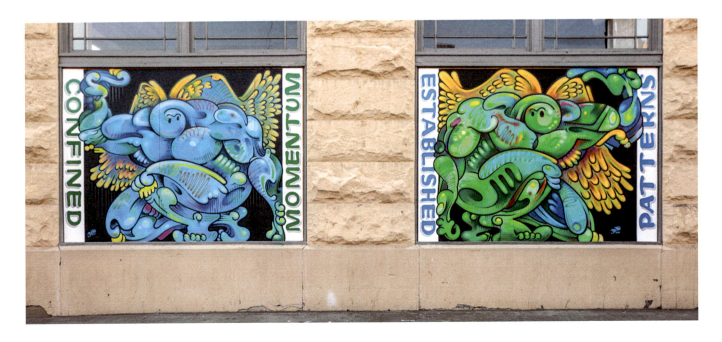

Photos: ARTIST

Artist:	Jay Mason
Name of Mural:	*She is Essential*
Materials:	Acrylic and oil on wood
Size:	8 x 6 feet
Location:	Flatstick Pub, 240 2nd Ave S
Coordinated by:	Alliance for Pioneer Square, Sara Pizzo, Public Realm Manager
Artist's website:	jaymasonart.com

"I painted this as a salute to women in the medical field on the front lines of the pandemic. The woman in my piece honors all of the women before her and all the women after her. She is Essential."

—Jay Mason

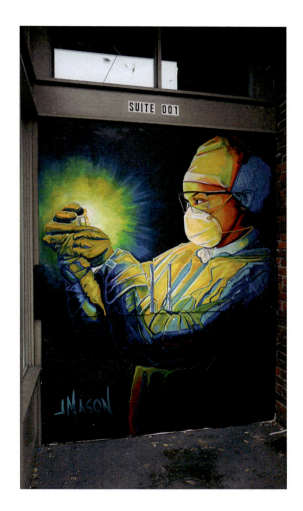

Photos: ARTIST

Artist:	Jay Mason
Name of Mural:	*Waiting with Paco*
Materials:	Acrylic and oils on wood
Size:	6 x 25 feet
Location:	Flat Stick Pub, 240 2nd Ave S
Coordinated by:	Sara Pizzo
Artist's website:	jaymasonart.com

"During the COVID-19 crisis, we spend a lot of time in our homes pondering when we will be able to return to our normal lives and what that new normal will look like. Waiting with Paco *captures that. It depicts Brandy King-Mason (my wife) and our dog, Paco, peering out a window at the city of Seattle, waiting for a time when COVID-19 is behind us so we can safely re-enter the world again."*

—Jay Mason

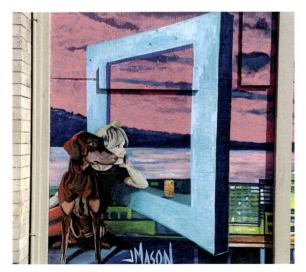 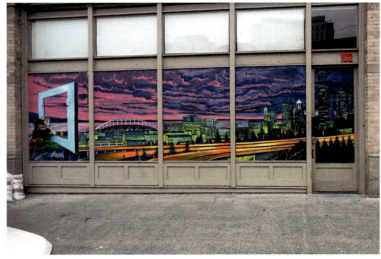

Photos: JEAN SHERRARD

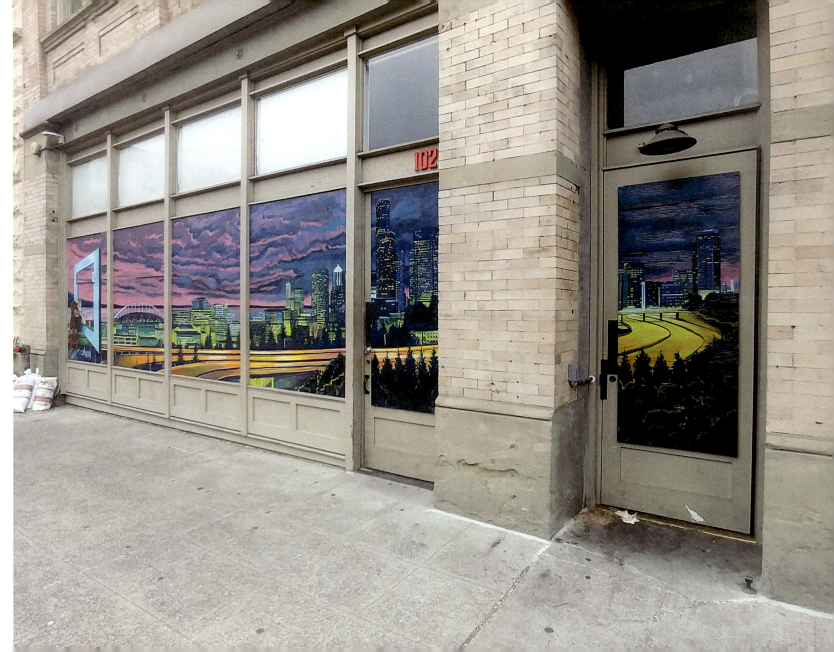

Artist: Joe Nix
Name of Mural: *Assemblage*
Materials: Latex, aerosol
Size: 8 x 26 feet
Location: Good Bar, 240 2nd Ave S
Coordinated by: Dom Nieri
Artist's website: @joe.nix on Instagram

"I painted the mural to help beautify the neighborhood."

—Joe Nix

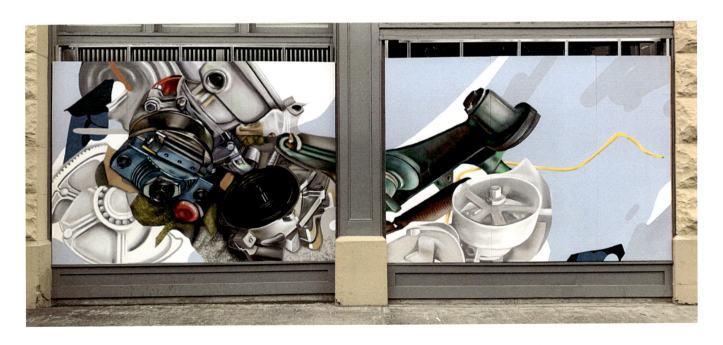

Photos: ARTIST

Artists: Lance Lobuzzetta / Efflux Creations
Name of Mural: *Winds of Change*
Materials: Spray paint, acrylic
Size: 8 x 11 feet
Location: Delmar Building, 118 1st Ave
Coordinated by: Alliance for Pioneer Square
Artist's website: Effluxcreations.com

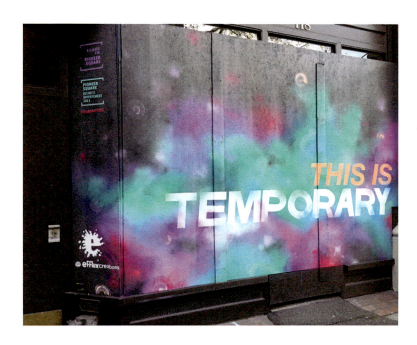

"Seemingly overnight, we transformed an eerily quiet and bleak scene into colorful streets filled with art. Rarely does an opportunity exist when artists get to come together to paint an entire neighborhood and be a part of a cohesive community message of hope. Amidst this crazy time, getting to contribute a little beauty and a positive mantra to a neighborhood that I love was just what I needed."

—Lance Lobuzzetta

Photos: ARTIST

Artist: Jonathan Wakuda Fischer
Name of Mural: *Rise Again*
Materials: Spray paint
Size: 7 x 45 feet
Location: ArtXchange Gallery, 512 1st Ave S
Artist's website: artxchange.org/artist/jonathan-wakuda-fischer

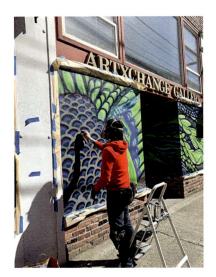 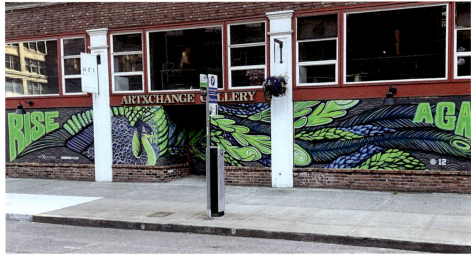

Photos: CORA EDMONDS

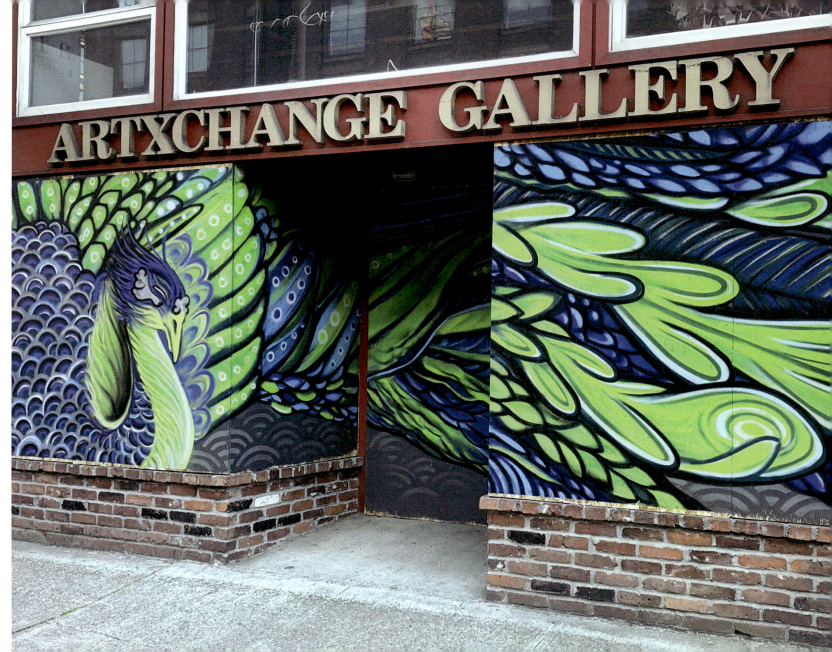

Artists:	Leo Shallat, Vladimir Kovalik
Name of Mural:	*This Too Shall Pass*
Materials:	Acrylic, aerosol, ink
Size:	10 x 28 feet
Location:	Emerald City Guitars, 83 S Washington St
Coordinated by:	Alliance for Pioneer Square
Artist's website:	Leoshallat.com, vksigns.com

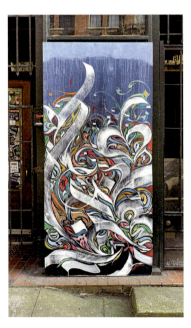 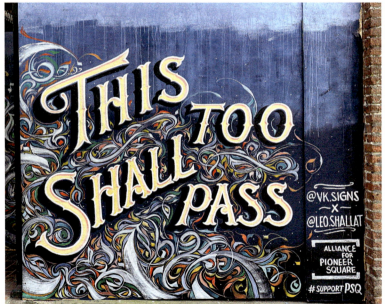

Photos: ARTIST

Artist:	Mason Montgomery
Name of Mural:	*Golden Dragon*
Materials:	Spray paint
Size:	12 x 10 feet
Location:	Altstadt Bierhalle & Brathaus, 209 1st Ave S
Coordinated by:	Overall Creative
Artist's website:	Moonlighttattooseattle.com

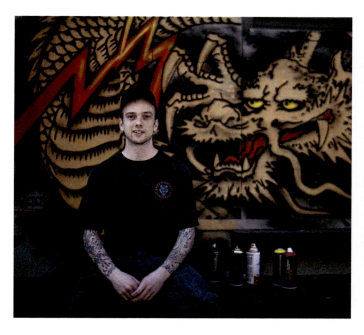 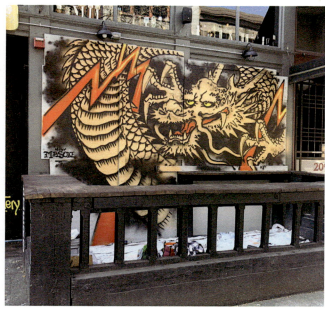

Photos: ARTIST, AUSTIN WILSON

Artist:	Mari Shibuya
Name of Mural:	*Creativity Regenerates*
Materials:	Exterior latex, acrylic, aerosol, love
Size:	9 x 15 feet
Location:	Vacant storefront, 220 1st Ave S
Coordinated by:	Jonathan "Wakuda" Fischer
Artist's website:	marishibuya.com

"This mural was a passion piece for me. I am deeply passionate about the healing, regenerative power of creativity at the individual and collective levels. I depicted a lush forest growing out of the arms of a dancing figure to express how our creativity is part of the expression of the creativity of the natural world. In this time of collapse, access to our own personal creativity and incentivizing our collective creativity will be crucial to our survival."

—Mari Shibuya

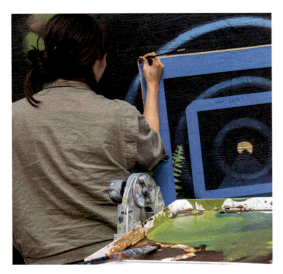 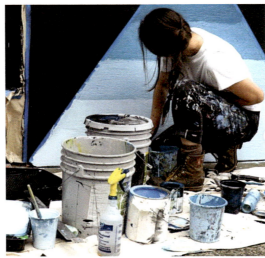

Photos: JORDAN SOMERS, GILLIAN PECKHAM

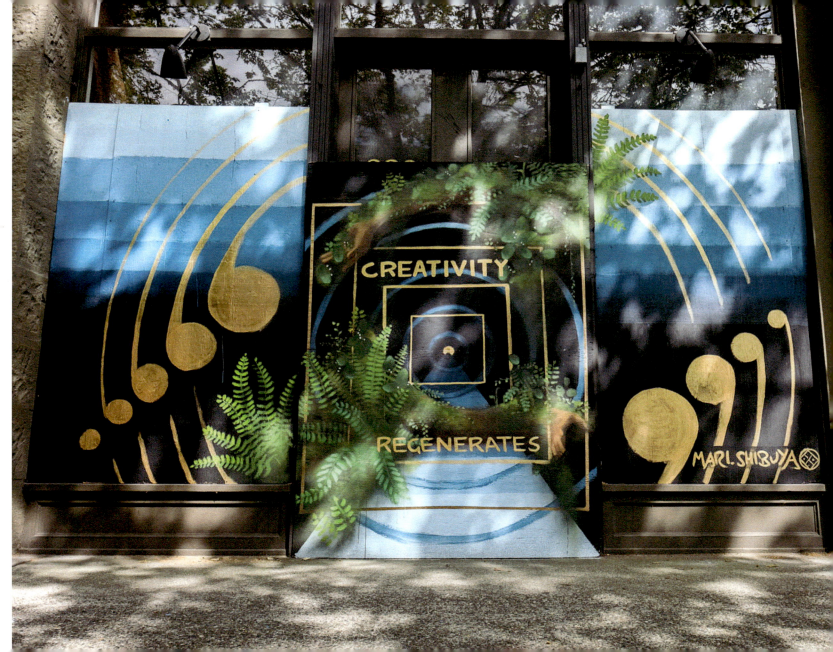

Artist:	Paul Nunn
Name of Mural:	*Wave to a Stranger*
Materials:	House paint, spray paint, acrylic paint
Size:	8 x 40 feet
Location:	Buttnick Building vacant storefront SE
Artist's website:	paulnunn.party

"I moved to Pioneer Square in mid-April. I had never lived in the city and was excited to get out of the house and in on the mural painting action. I started asking around to get permission when I saw other artists working and was lucky enough to connect with the right people to do the work."

—Paul Nunn

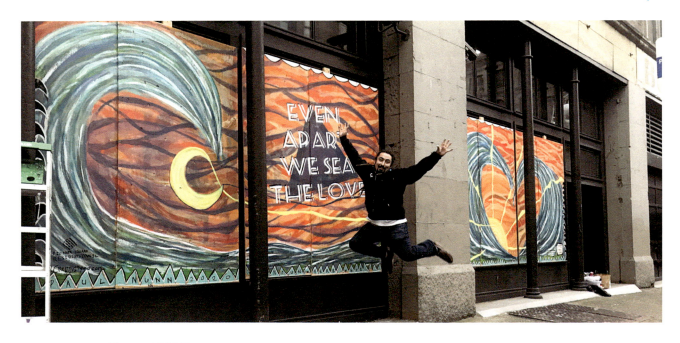

Photos: ARTIST

Artist: Paul Nunn
Name of Mural: *Non-Sequi-Doors*
Materials: Stencils, spraypaint
Size: 5 x 2 feet each
Location: Buttnick Building vacant storefront
Artist's website: paulnunn.party

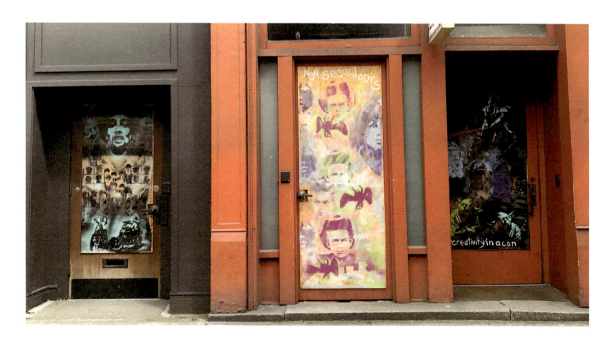

Photos: ARTIST

Artist:	Ray Monde
Name of Mural:	*Together Apart*
Materials:	*Seattle Times*, wheatpaste, paint
Size:	8 x 56 feet
Location:	Swannie's Sports Bar, 109 S Washington St
Coordinated by:	Sara Pizzo
Credits:	"Seattle's Poem" by Claudia Castro Luna
Artist's website:	raymonde.com.au

"I really wanted to create something to keep people's spirits up. I wanted us all to be able to look on the bright side—even though we're locked inside and can't see the people we love— we can still be part of the incredible natural beauty all around us. I really love how Seattle pulled together to get through this."

—Ray Monde

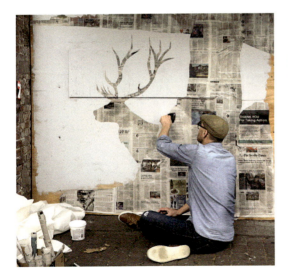
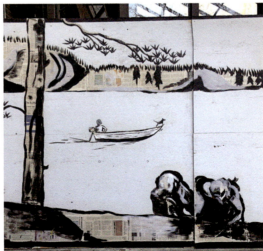
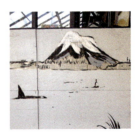

Photos: CHRIS KIRBY

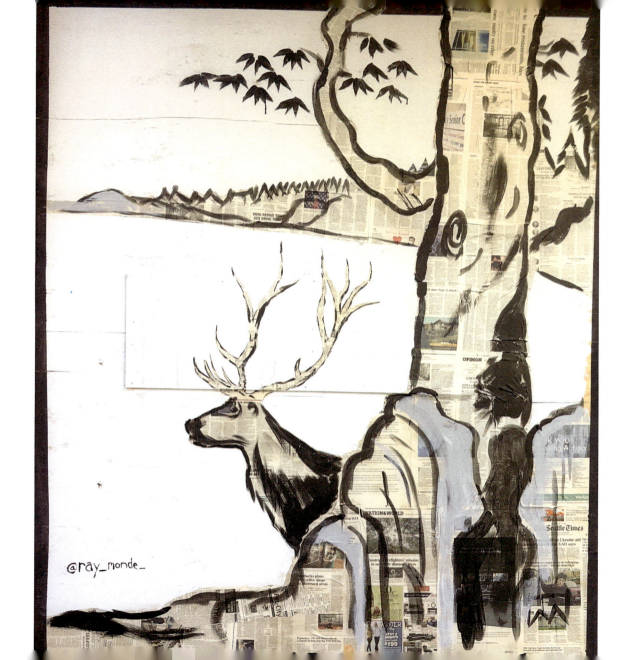

Artist: Sam Day
Name of Mural: *Globe Bookstore Mural*
Materials: Acrylic paint
Size: 8 x 16 feet
Location: Globe Bookstore, 218 1st Ave S
Coordinated by: Joe Siscoe
Artist's website: samday.com

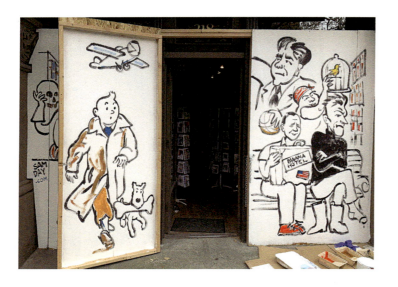

"When the plywood went up around Pioneer Square, I suggested this mural to John Siscoe, owner of The Globe Bookstore, with whom I have been friends for many years. A bookstore is a place of a thousand personalities, but I only had room for a dozen."

—Sam Day

Photos: ARTIST

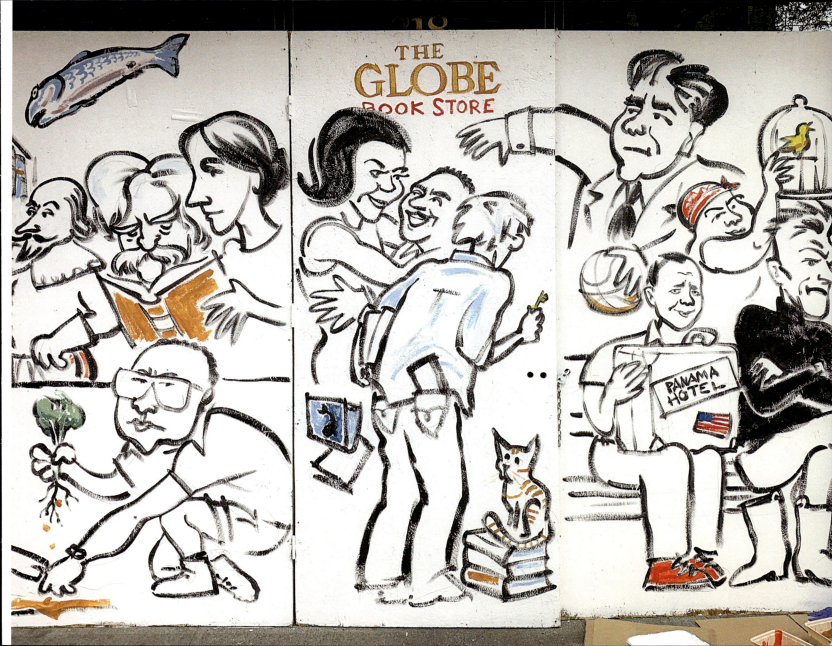

Artist:	Sydney M. Pertl
Crew:	Miles Pertl, Leah Terada, SeaPertl Productions
Name of Mural:	*Be Sure to Wash Your Flippers—Duck, Duck, Duck...*
Materials:	House paints, sharpies, love, memories
Size:	9 x 15 feet and 8 x 16 feet
Location:	Agate Designs, 102 1st Ave S
Coordinated by:	Sara Pizzo
Artist's website:	sydneympertl.com, seapertls.com

"*I am not a healthcare worker or grocery store employee, and, as the world was shutting down around me, I struggled to see how I could contribute or help. This project has given me a way to use my skills and talents to do my part for Seattle; I am using my artwork to bring hope and joy to my city throughout these trying times.*"

—Sydney M. Pertl

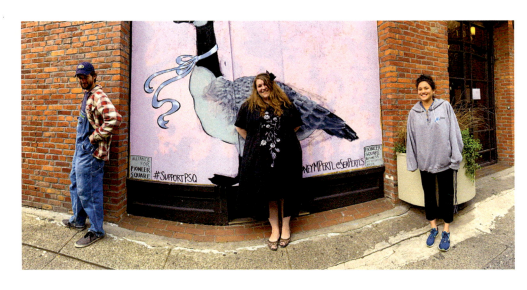

Photos: ARTIST, MILES PERTL

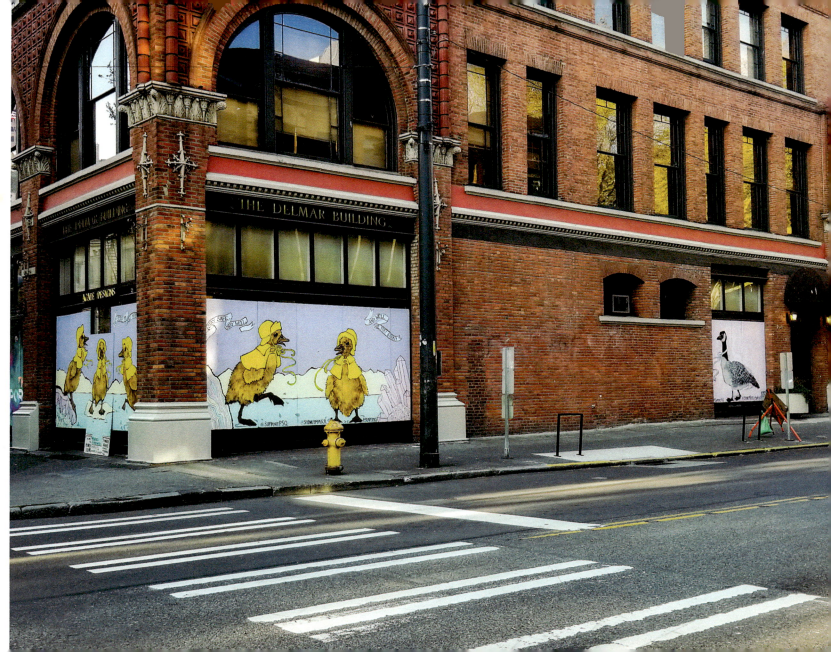

Artist:	Tara Velan
Name of Mural:	*Slow Jam*
Materials:	Exterior paint
Size:	8 x 36 feet
Location:	Buttnick Building LP, 206 1st Ave S
Artist's website:	@yesitstara on Instagram

"We artists came together as a collective to protect the buildings, encourage Seattle, and let everyone know we are in this together. This experience sealed the deal that Seattle is home—and that creatives still exist here with something to say. I am so grateful to have been a part of this movement."

—Tara Velan

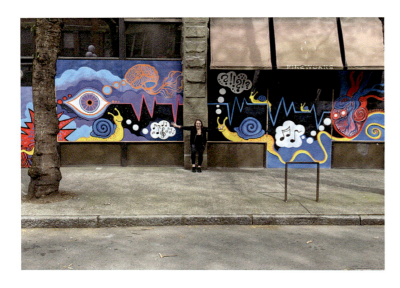

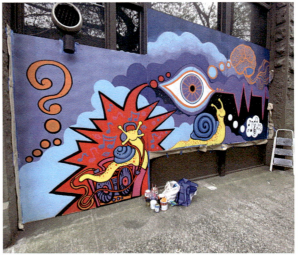

Photos: ARTIST

Artists: Vladimir Kovalik, Leo Shallat
Name of Mural: *Wish You Were Here*
Materials: Spray paint, acrylic
Size: 8 x 20 feet
Location: The Central Saloon, 207 1st Ave S
Artist's website: vksigns.com

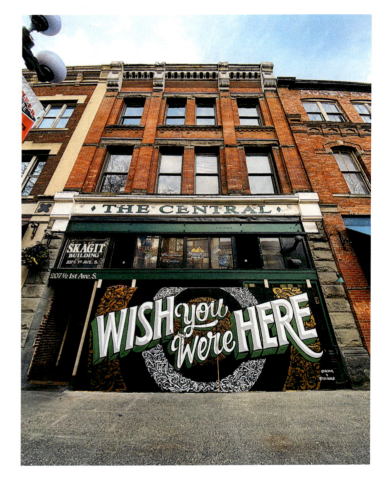

Photos: MANDEE RAE

Artists:	Zaeos
Name of Mural:	*Ebony Beauty*
Materials:	Spray paint and latex
Size:	7 x 12 feet
Location:	formerly J&M Cafe, 201 1st Ave S
Coordinated by:	Overall Creative
Artist's website:	@zaeos on Instagram

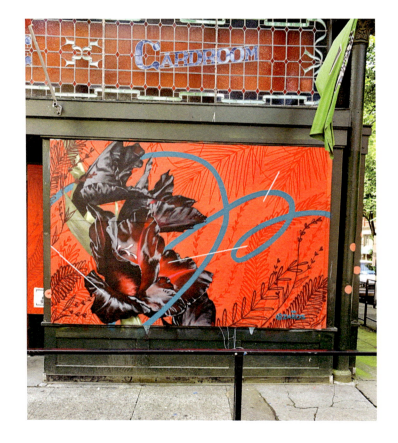

48   **Photos:** ARTIST

Downtown

Artist: Ariel Parrow
Name of Mural: *Jasper, Chubbs Peterson, Trout, Gus, and Ruby*
Materials: Acrylics
Size: 8 x 14 feet
Location: Palihotel, 107 Pine St
Coordinated by: Seth Geiser, Downtown Seattle Cares
Artist's website: thechaoticaquatic.com

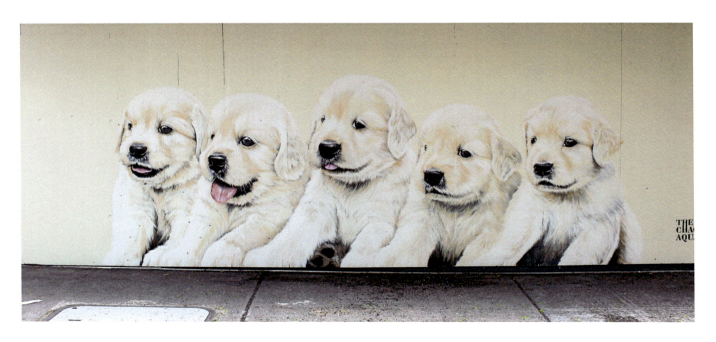

Photos: ARTIST

Artist:	Burgandy Viscosi
Name of Mural:	*Healthy Lungs* (series)
Materials:	Acrylic
Size:	varied
Locations:	Re-Bar, 1114 Howell st
	Devil's Triangle, 2027 Westlake Ave
	Showgirls, 1510 1st Ave
Artist's website:	Burgandyviscosi.com

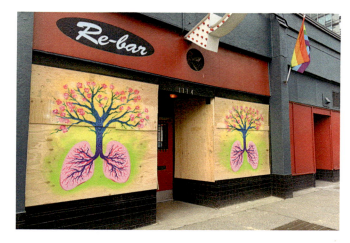

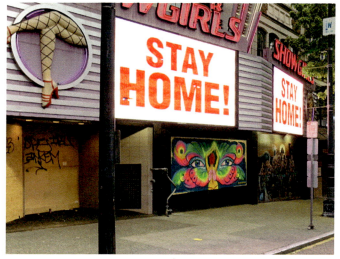

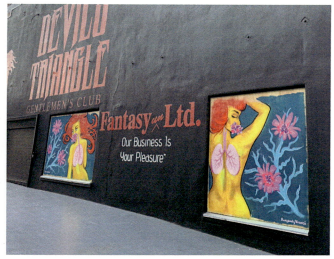

Photos: ARTIST

Artist:	Devon Midori Hale
Name of Mural:	*Toujours Café Campagne (Café Campagne Forever)*
Materials:	Latex paints
Size:	8 x 48 feet
Location:	Café Campagne, 1600 Post Alley
Artist's website:	devonmidorihale.com

"Prior to the coronavirus shutdown, I was a server at Café Campagne. When I lost my job in March, I was also mourning the identity and culture built within the restaurant industry, which seemed to disintegrate all at once. As a muralist in food service, I painted to reestablish my connection to a job I miss and to create a positive visual for the Pike Place Market neighborhood, which has been hit particularly hard by this crisis. I borrowed from French Impressionism to envision a future return of restaurant life, with new norms—takeout, eating outdoors, physical distancing—while never diminishing the timeless importance and beauty of enjoying a good meal with those we love."

—Devon Hale

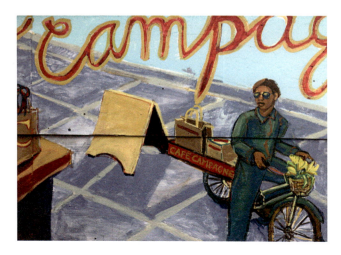
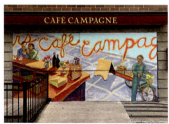
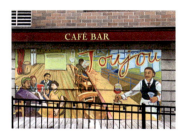

Photos: ARTIST

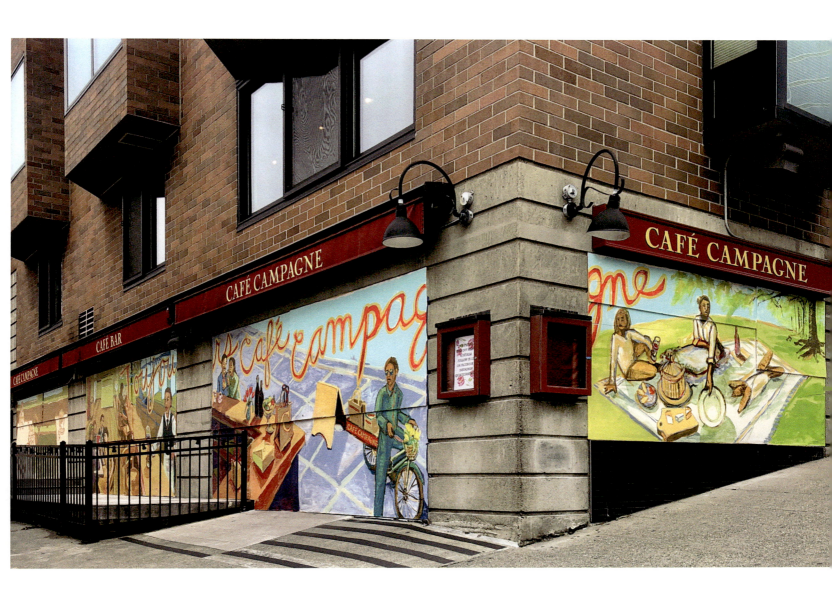

Artists:	Dozfy
Name of Mural:	*Meat*
Materials:	Latex, enamel, acrylic paint
Size:	10 x 20 each
Location:	Metropolitan Grill, 820 2nd Ave
Coordinated by:	Nicole Alyn
Artist's website:	Dozfy.net

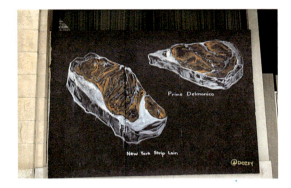

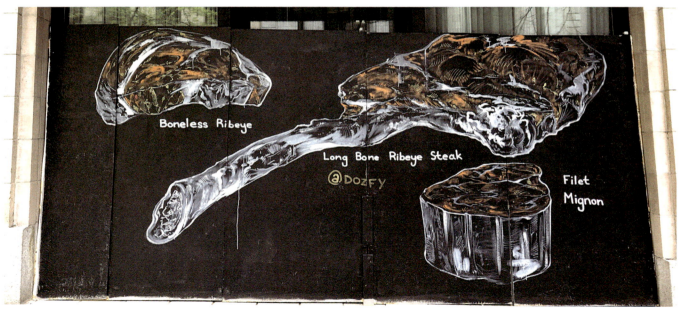

54   Photos: ARTIST

Artist:	Dozfy	*Stay Strong Reflection*
Name of Mural:	*Untitled*	
Materials:	Latex, acrylic paint	Latex, aerosol, acrylic paint, mirror
Size:	8 x 8 feet	4 x 10 feet
Location:	Sneaker City, 110 Pike St	Some Random Bar, 2604 1st Avenue
Coordinated by:	Caroline Cho	Michael Maione, Brian Lee
Artist's website:	Dozfy.net	Dozfy.net

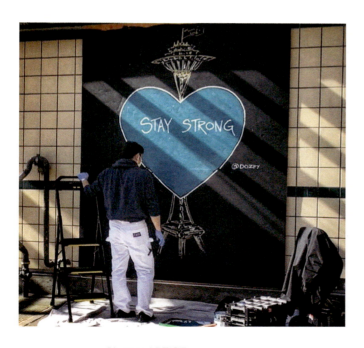
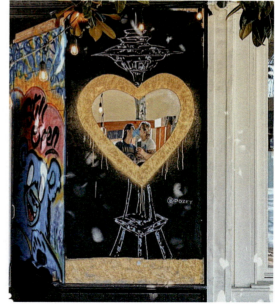

Photos: ARTIST

Artist: Dillon Bennett
Name of Mural: *Untitled*
Materials: Interior house paint, primer, plywood
Size: 9 x 8 feet
Location: STT Lettering, 2232 1st Ave S
Coordinated by: Lauren Ross
Artist's website: dillonbennettart.com

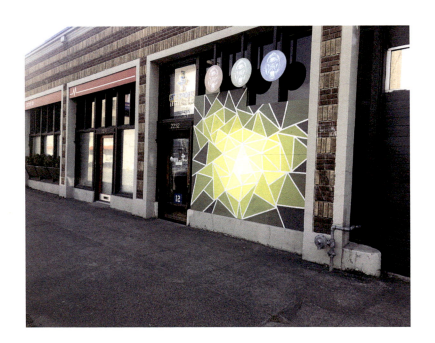

56   **Photos:** LAUREN ROSS

Artist: Sandy
Name of Mural: *Barefeet on Scare St.*
Materials: Rustoleum and Montana paint on latex
Size: 10 x 20 feet
Location: Nordstrom, 500 Pine St
Coordinated by: Urban Artworks
Artist's website: @paint_2_change on Instagram

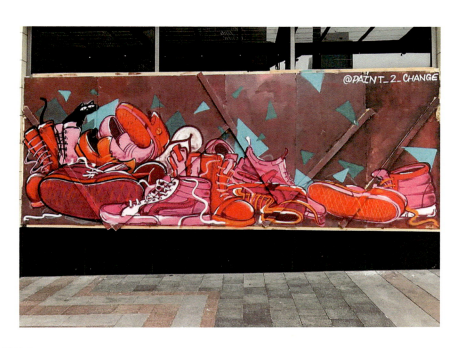

Photos: NOT ORANGES MURALS

Artist: Sarah Robbins
Crew: Christina Dean and Jessica Cantwell
Name of Mural: *Just Keep Going*
Materials: Latex paint
Size: 8 x 8 feet and 8 x 15 ft
Location: McDonalds, 1530 3rd Ave
Coordinated by: Downtown Seattle Association
Artist's website: sarah-robbins.com

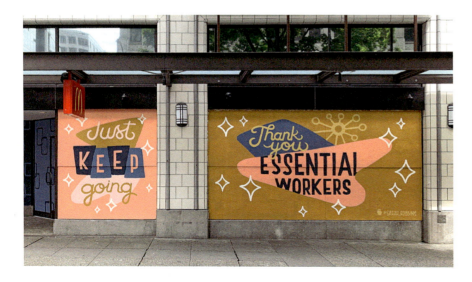

Photos: ARTIST

Artists:	Sarah Robbins
Crew:	Christina Dean and Jessica Cantwell
Name of Mural:	*Call Your Mom*
Materials:	Latex paint
Size:	8 x 18 feet
Location:	McDonald's, 1530 3rd Ave
Coordinated by:	Downtown Seattle Association
Artist's website:	sarah-robbins.com

"I am honored to be a part of that movement. These frightening and uncertain times are impacting each one of us differently and a lot of people are looking for ways to help. The least I can do is throw some paint up on a few boards around town to try and make someone's day a teeny bit brighter. Art is powerful, and in these times it can act as a reminder that we are here to help each other, and that we will get through this together. Here's hoping these messages remind you to stay positive, stay safe, and above all else, call your mom."

—Sarah Robbins

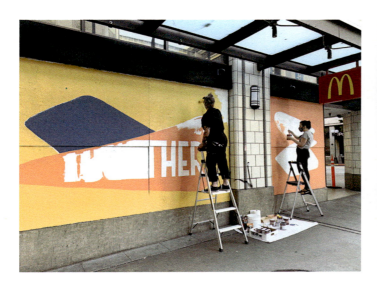
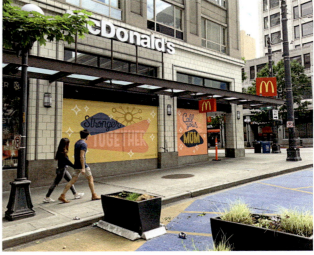

Photos: ARTIST

59

Artists:	Joanna Fitzgerald, Sabrina Prestes
Crew:	Sophia Oliveira
Name of Mural:	*Resilience*
Materials:	Acrylic on wood
Size:	8 x 20 feet
Location:	Old Navy, 511 Pine St
Artist's website:	@illustrationbyjoanna on Instagram

"I decided to paint this mural in order to encourage people that, like cacti, we can be resilient and survive even in the most difficult conditions. My goal was to spark beauty and joy in the downtown area."

—Joanna Fitzgerald

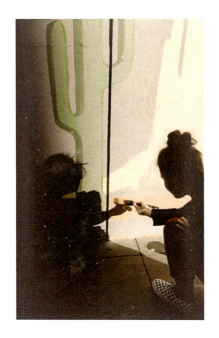 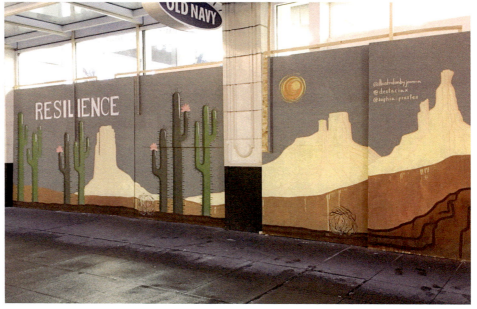

Photos: ARTISTS

Belltown

Artists:	Billie Avery
Crew:	Kimberly Tieu
Name of Mural:	*Together We Stand*
Materials:	Paint
Size:	7 x 10 feet
Location:	Rudy's Barbershop, 89 Wall St
Coordinated by:	Overall Creative
Artist's website:	Therirualartist.com

"Mural painting has been an aspiration of mine for many years, and I was inspired to finally do one by the mural projects that have been covering the streets of Seattle during the COVID-19 pandemic, uplifting our community. As a queer person, I wanted to create a piece that demonstrated the unity of our intersectional LGBTQ+ community during this crisis."

—Billie Avery

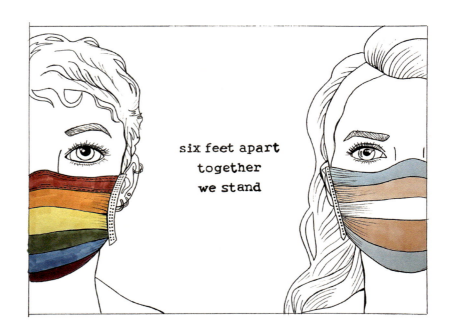

Photos: ARTIST

Artist:	Burgandy Viscosi
Name of Mural:	*Healthy Lungs* (series)
Materials:	Acrylic
Size:	varied
Locations:	Seahorse Bar, 2201 1st Ave
	City Hostel, 2327 2nd Ave
	Belltown Pizza, 2422 1st Ave
Artist's website:	burgandyviscosi.com

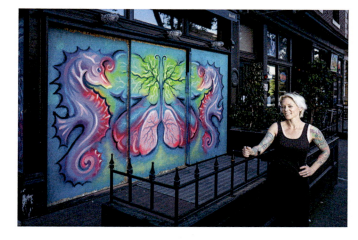

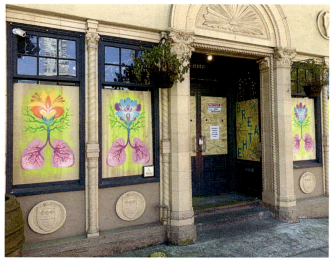

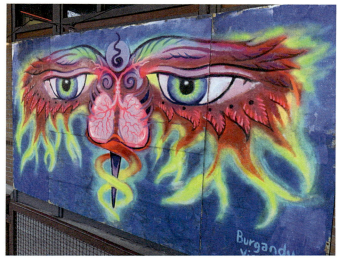

Photos: ARTIST

Artist: Dozfy
Name of Mural: *Orcas*
Materials: Latex, oil and acrylic paint
Size: 8 x 8 feet each
Location: The Virginia Inn, 1937 1st Ave
Coordinated by: Karl Sexton
Artist's website: Dozfy.net

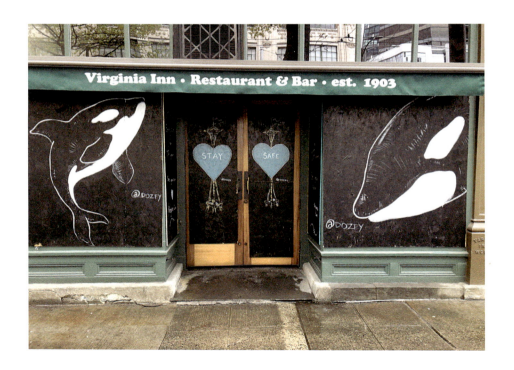

Photos: ARTIST

Artist:	Dozfy	
Name of Mural:	*Epic battle*	*Seahorse*
Materials:	Latex, oil and acyrlic paint	Latex, oil and acrylic paint
Size:	12 x 20 feet	4 x 6 feet
Location:	Amber Seattle, 2214 1st Avenue	Seahorse Bar, 2201 1st Avenue
Coordinated by:	Michael Jerrett	Linda Derschang
Artist's website:	Dozfy.net	Dozfy.net

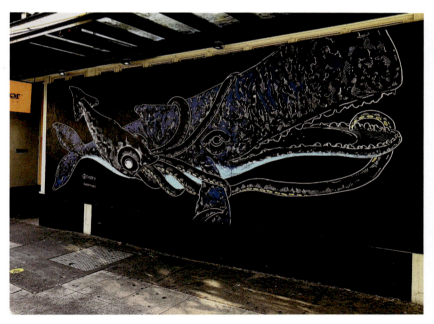
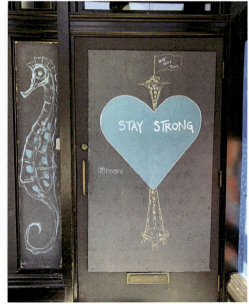

Photos: ARTIST

Artist:	Dozfy
Name of Mural:	*Heartwood*
Materials:	Latex, enamel, acrylic paint
Size:	30 x 10 feet
Location:	Heartwood Provisions, 1103 1st Ave
Coordinated by:	Nicole Alyn
Artist's website:	Dozfy.net

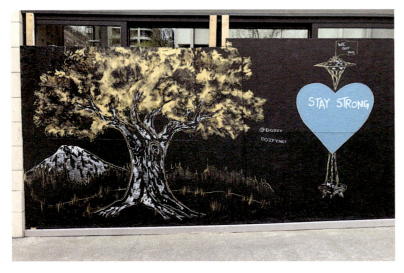

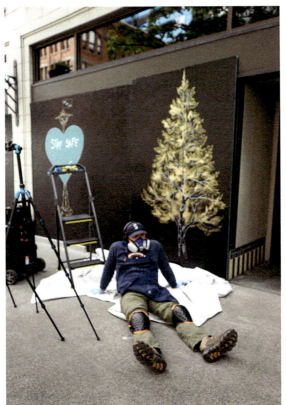

66   Photos: ARTIST

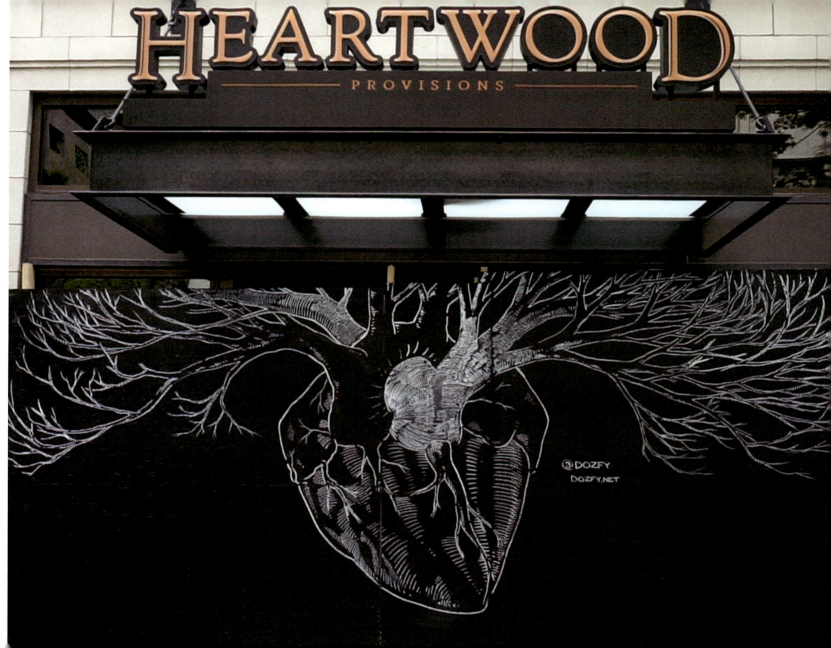

Artist:	Dozfy	
Name of Mural:	*Stay Strong*	*Untitled*
Materials:	Latex, oil and acrylic paint	Latex Paint
Size:	4 x 8 feet	8 x 10 feet
Location:	Belltown Pizza, 2422 1st Ave	Harris Harvey Gallery, 1915 1st Ave
Coordinated by:	Michael Jerrett	Linda Derschang
Artist's website:	Dozfy.net	Dozfy.net

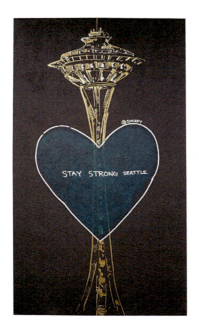
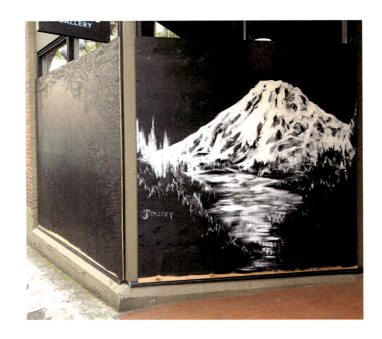

68   Photos: ARTIST

Artists: Sandy
Name of Mural: *Sandy's Garage*
Materials: Rustoleum and latex
Size: 9 x 12 feet
Location: Amber Seattle, 2214 1st Ave
Coordinated by: Dozfy
Artist's website: @paint_2_change on Instagram

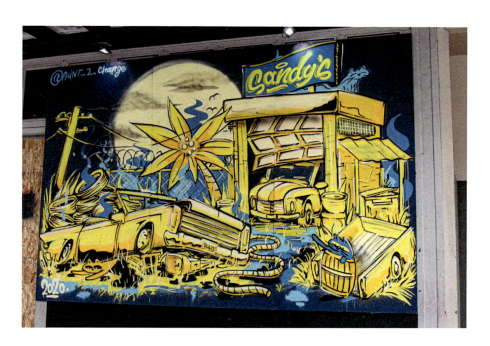

Photos: MATTHEW MACDONALD

Artists: Lina Cholewinski, Rob Tardiff
Name of Mural: *Floral Daydream*
Materials: Spray paint, acrylic
Size: 15 x 30 feet
Location: Vue Lounge, 2324 2nd Ave
Coordinated by: Overall Creative
Credits: model: Kelsey Allen
Artist's website: @bonesandgold, @zaeos on Instagram

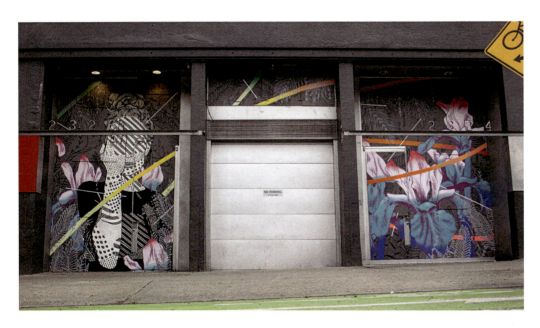

Photos: AUSTIN WILSON

Artists:	Shavonne Maes
Name of Mural:	*Imagine*
Materials:	Spray paint, acrylic, glitter.
Size:	3 x 5 feet
Location:	Some Random Bar, 2604 1st Ave
Coordinated by:	Brian Lee, Belltown Pizza
Credits:	John Lennon (text of quote)
Artist's website:	@oramiorigami on Instagram

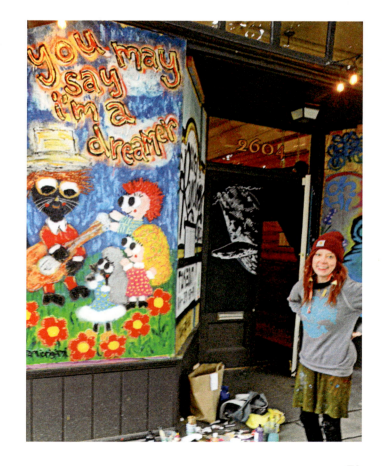

"My amazing cat Fern has been my inspiration and gotten me through all of my dark times. People ask about her everyday. Oh Fern!"

—Shavonne Maes

Photos: CATHARINE ANISTETT

Artist:	Tara Velan
Name of Mural:	*Finding _____ .*
Materials:	Exterior paint
Size:	6 x 4 feet
Location:	Queen City, 2201 1st Ave
Coordinated by:	Linda Derschang
Credits:	Linda Derschang and Brian Lee
Artist's website:	@yesitstara on Instagram

Pizzacorn

Acrylic paint

5 x 10 feet

Belltown Pizza, 2422 1st Ave

Brian Lee

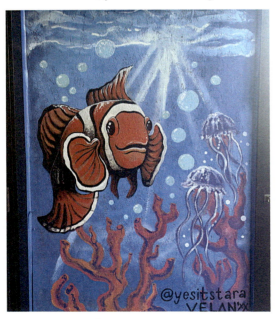

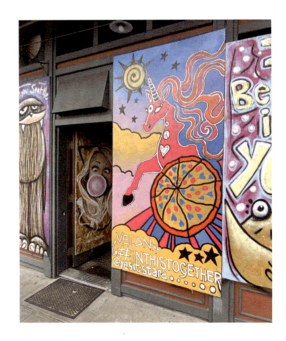

Photos: ARTIST

Capitol Hill

Artist: Amanda Joyce Bishop
Crew: Rosie Alyea
Name of Mural: *Purple Moonscape*
Materials: Latex paint, enamel, plywood
Size: 12 x 4 feet
Location: Comet Tavern, 922 E Pike St
Coordinated by: Overall Creative
Artist's website: @purebonaventure on Instagram

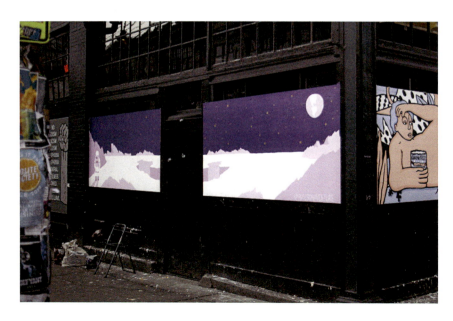

Photos: AUSTIN WILSON

Artist: Ariel Parrow
Name of Mural: *Float On*
Materials: Acrylic house paint
Size: 5 x 8 feet
Location: Lost Lake Cafe, 1505 10th Ave
Coordinated by: Kathleen Warren, Overall Creative
Artist's website: thechaoticaquatic.com

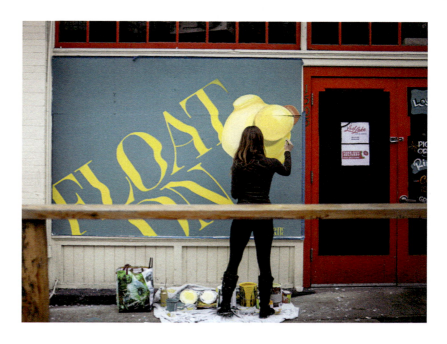

Photos: AUSTIN WILSON

Artist:	Anne Siems
Crew:	Kathleen Warren of Overallcreative, Camillo Massagli
Name of Mural:	*Beauty + Terror*
Materials:	Acrylic paint, house paint
Size:	8 x 20 feet
Location:	Life on Mars, 722 E Pike St
Coordinated by:	Kathleen Warren of Overall Creative
Credits:	Rainer Maria Rilke for use of lines of his poem, "Go to the Limits of your Longing"
Artist's website:	annesiems.com

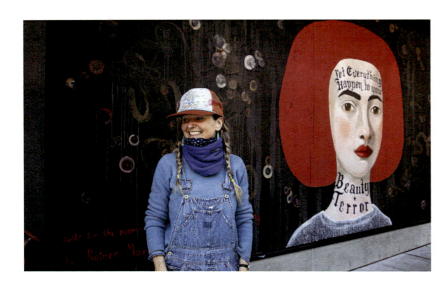

Photos: AUSTIN WILSON

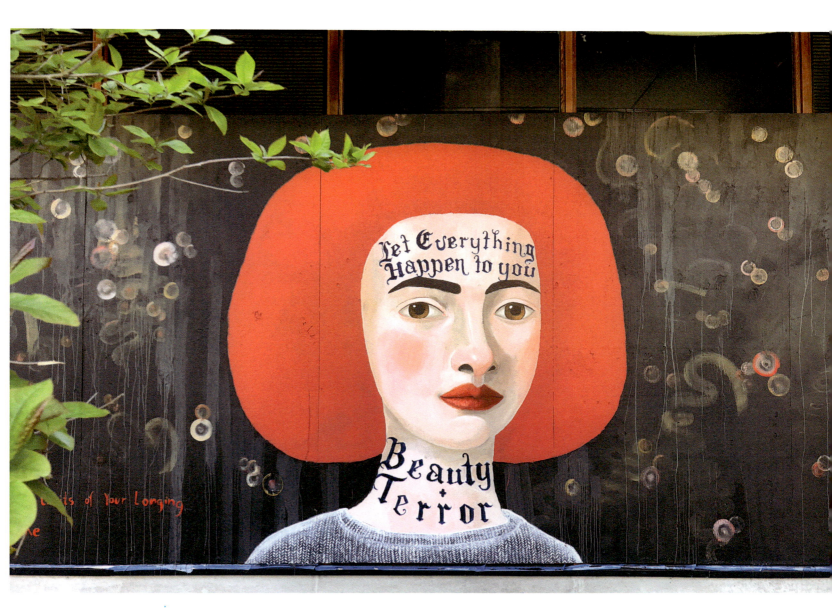

Artist: AxeHAKA
Name of Mural: *Untitled*
Materials: Custom stencil, latex paint
Size: 8 x 6 feet
Location: Ritual, 914 E Pike St
Artist's website: facedowncraftsup.com

"Ritual asked the local artists they feature to do art not only to promote ourselves, but also to do what we love: creepy dolls! I chose to use this stencil of one of my doll photos as I usually work in 3D Mixed Media Art form."

—AxeHAKA

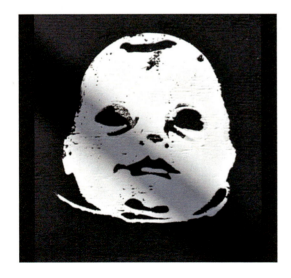 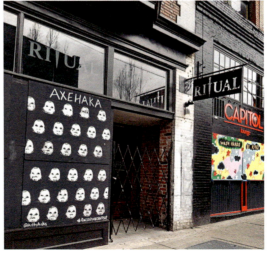

Photos: LADYHAKA, SARAH WILLIAMS, ROXANN MURRAY

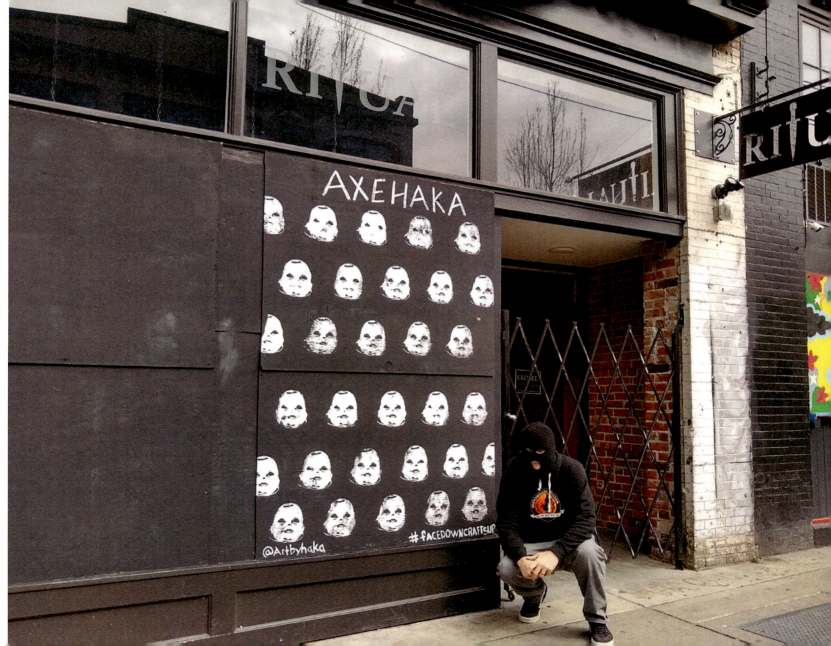

Artist: C.M. Ruiz
Name of Mural: *Miriam*
Materials: Xerox, wheatpaste, ink
Size: 6 x 8 feet
Location: Linda's Tavern, 707 E Pine St
Artist's website: cmruiz.com

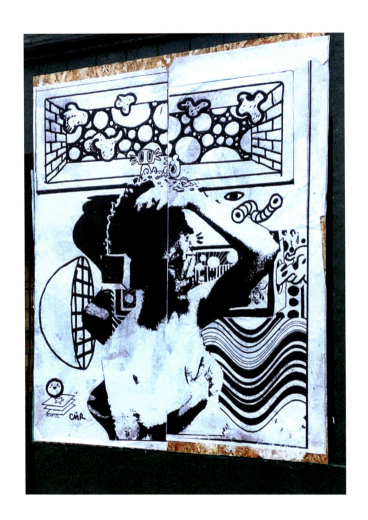

"Linda's is one of my favorite bars, so I wanted to help bring art to their building during the coronavirus shutdown. I used my background in street art and wheatpasting to do this project.."

—C.M. Ruiz

80   Photos: ARTIST

Artists:	Cady Bogart
Name of Mural:	*Quarantine Cutie*
Materials:	House paint, wood panel
Size:	4 x 8 feet
Location:	The Comet Tavern, 922 E Pike St
Coordinated by:	Overall Creative
Credits:	Kathleen Warren for her help prepping and priming
Artist's website:	cadybogart.com

"I chose the design of somebody lounging and snacking because it was something light-hearted and relatable to everyone at the time of making the mural. At a time of so much uncertainty and worry for a lot of people, I wanted to make something that could be enjoyed through laughter."

—Cady Bogart

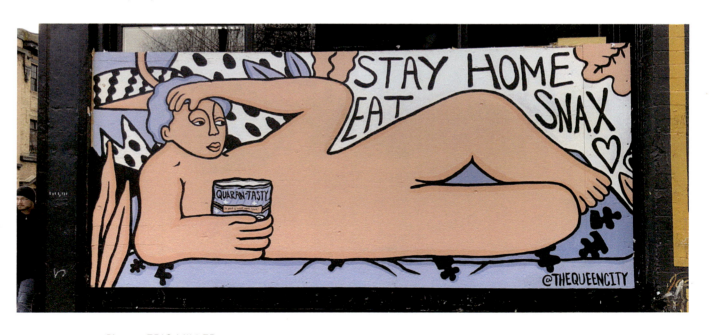

Photos: ERIC MILLER

Artist:	Casey Weldon
Crew:	Crystal Barbre
Name of Mural:	*We Will Land on Our Feet*
Materials:	Acrylics, oils
Size:	6 x 10 feet
Location:	Roq La Rue, 705 E Pike St
Artist's website:	caseyweldon.com, crystalbarbre.com

"When businesses first started boarding up their storefronts, Crystal and I got to talking about what a shame it was to see all of this ugly plywood. We wondered if any of the businesses would be interested in letting us decorate them. When one of our favorite galleries, Roq La Rue, posted their newly boarded up windows, I immediately contacted Kirsten and asked if she would do us the honor of allowing us to beautify a local business that has brought so much beauty to us. It was the least we could do! "

—Casey Weldon

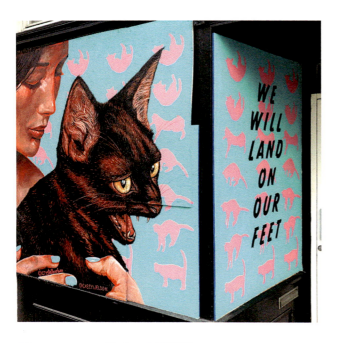

Photos: ARTISTS

Artist: Dozfy
Name of Mural: *Untitled*
Materials: Latex, oil, acrylic paint
Size: 10 x 18 feet
Location: Adana, 1449 E Pine St
Coordinated by: Adana (Shota and Alex)
Artist's website: Dozfy.net

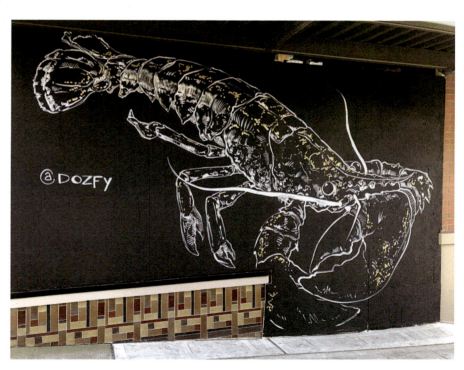

Photos: ARTIST

83

Artists:	Crystal Barbre, Casey Weldon
Crew:	Zach Takasawa
Name of Mural:	*Hello?*
Materials:	Acrylic, aerosol, latex, oils
Size:	8 x 20 feet
Location:	Life on Mars, 722 E Pike St
Coordinated by:	Overall Creative
Artist's website:	crystalbarbre.com, caseyweldon.com

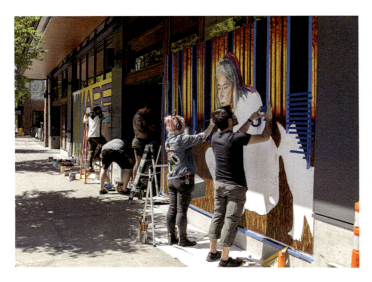 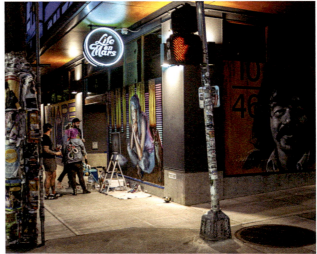

Photos: CASEY WELDEN, AUSTIN WILSON

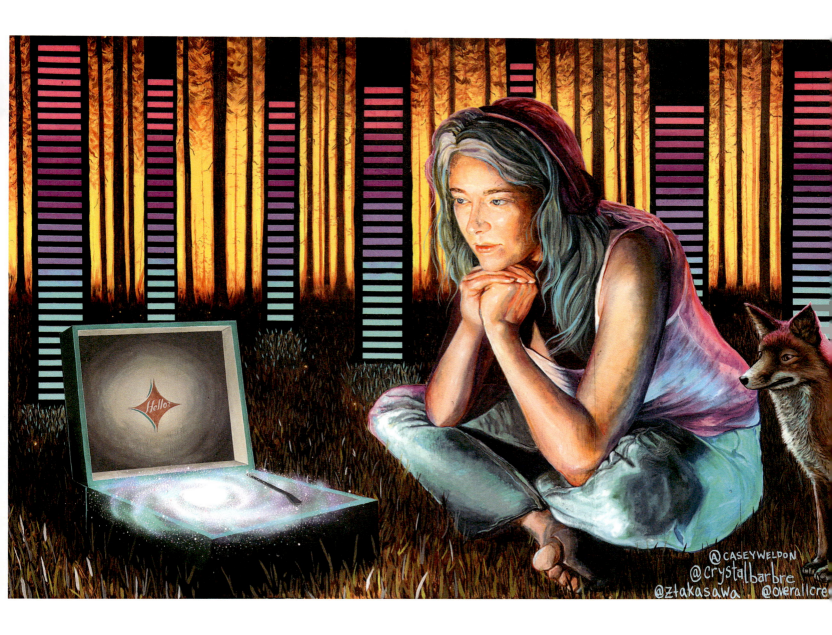

Artist: Burgandy Viscosi
Name of Mural: *Healthy Lungs* (series)
Materials: Acrylic
Size: 4 x 8 feet
Location: Retail Therapy, 905 E Pike St
Artist's website: Burgandyviscosi.com

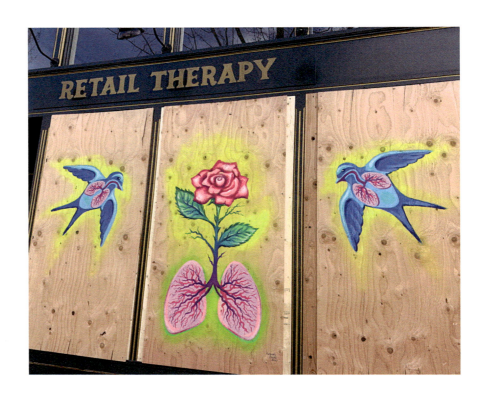

Photos: ARTIST

Artist:	Ethan Rivelle
Name of Mural:	*Keep Floating*
Materials:	Spray paint
Size:	4 x 12 feet
Location:	The Wild Rose, 1021 E Pike St
Coordinated by:	Sam Whitehead
Artist's website:	ethanrivelle.com

"I painted this mural to add some more positivity to the neighborhood and community during this uncertain time. It's a simple design, smiling faces of bubble characters I created. I was hoping if people saw the characters smiling it would put a smile on their faces too."

—Ethan Rivelle

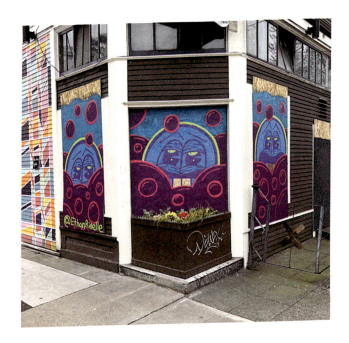

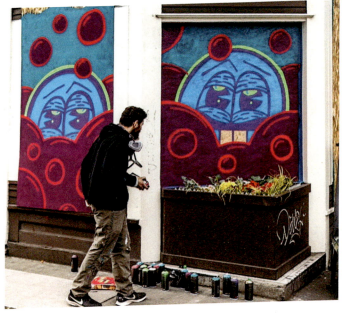

Photos: JAKE MILLETT

Artist: Evann Strathern
Name of Mural: *Sending Hugs From Afar*
Materials: Plywood, paint
Size: 12 x 10 feet
Location: Broadway Market Complex, 401 Broadway E
Coordinated by: Overall Creative
Artist's website: evann.com

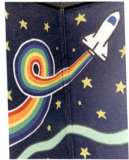

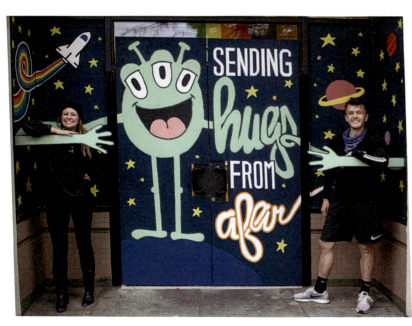

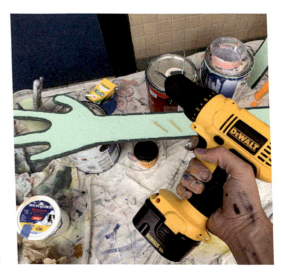

Photos: ARTIST, AUSTIN WILSON

Artists:	Ezra Dickinson
Name of Mural:	*YOU ARE NOT ALONE*
Materials:	Acrylic paint
Size:	8 x 20 feet
Location:	Life on Mars, 722 E Pike St
Coordinated by:	Kathleen Warren, Overall Creative
Credits:	John Richards, KEXP, and Michael Jackson
Artist's website:	EzraDickinson.com

"YOU ARE NOT ALONE is a profoundly human response that could be said to anyone at any time. I have always made gifts for my mother; I viewed this mural as an offering of intention for her and everyone."

—Ezra Dickinson

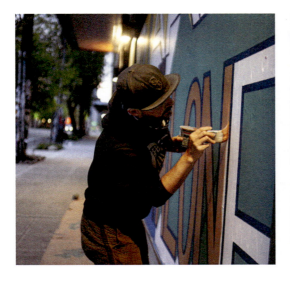 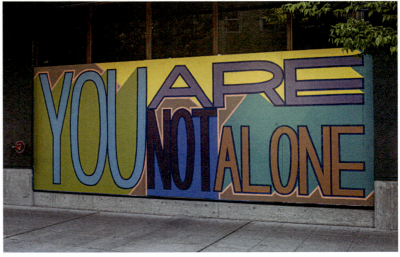

Photos: AUSTIN WILSON

89

Artist:	Goldsuit
Crew:	Genevieve St. Charles, Kevin Drake
Name of Mural:	*BE NICE*
Materials:	Spray paint
Size:	6 x 8 feet
Location:	Lost Lake, 1515 10th Ave
Coordinated by:	Kathleen Warren
Artist's website:	artofgoldsuit.com

"I wanted to contribute to the creation of a transformative, socially significant public art gallery in Capitol Hill. The BE NICE text is to remind people to be kind to each other during these volatile, difficult, and polarizing times."

—Goldsuit

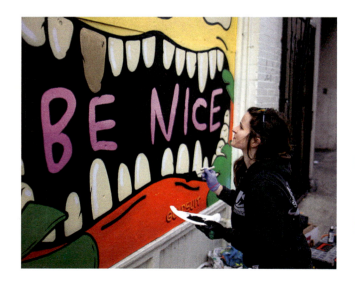 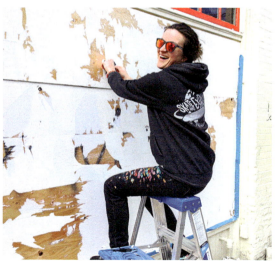

Photos: AUSTIN WILSON, KATHLEEN WARREN, GENEVIEVE ST. CHARLES

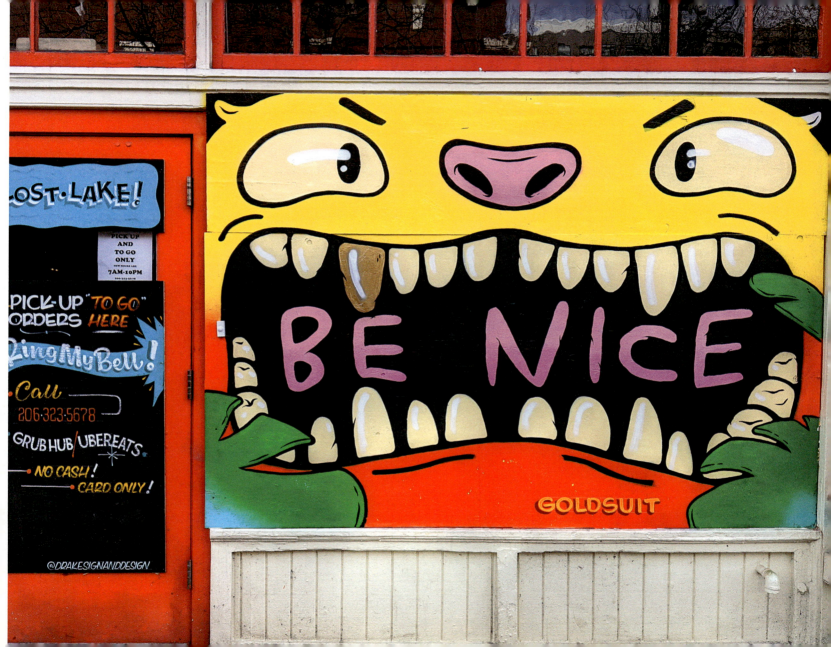

Artists:	Jake Millett
Name of Mural:	*Shine*
Materials:	House paint, spray paint, metallic ink
Size:	5.5 x 11 feet
Location:	Castle Megastore, 1017 E Pike St
Credits:	Maya Angelou (text of quote)
Artist's website:	jakemillett.com @bubzini on Instagram

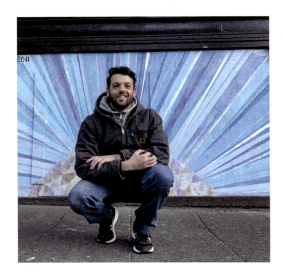 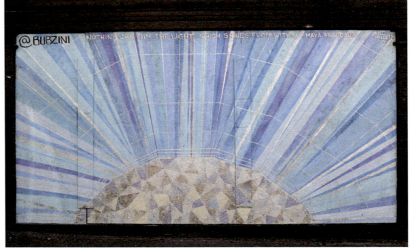

Photos: ARTIST

Artists: Jake Millett, Vladimir Kovalik
Crew: Hannah Gorder, Anna Josephson-Day
Name of Mural: *Call Yer Mom*
Materials: House paint, spray paint, acrylics, paint pens.
Size: 8 x 25 feet
Location: Urban Outfitters, 401 Broadway E
Coordinated by: Overall Creative
Artist's website: jakemillett.com, vksigns.com

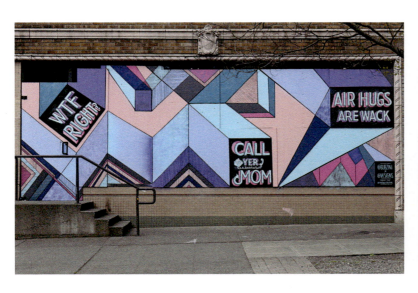

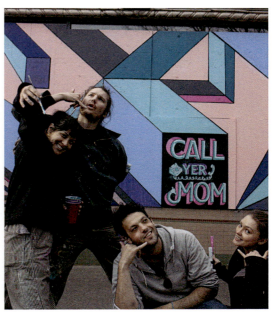

Photos: JAKE MILLET, AUSTIN WILSON

Artist: Jillian Chong
Name of Mural: *Seattle Strong*
Materials: Acrylic paint, spray paint, acrylic paint markers
Size: 8 x 19.5 feet
Location: Quinn's Pub, 1001 E Pike St
Artist's website: jillianchong.com

"I painted these murals because I saw it as an opportunity to help the community, get my work out there, and add some inspiration to the world in this dark time."

—Jillian Chong

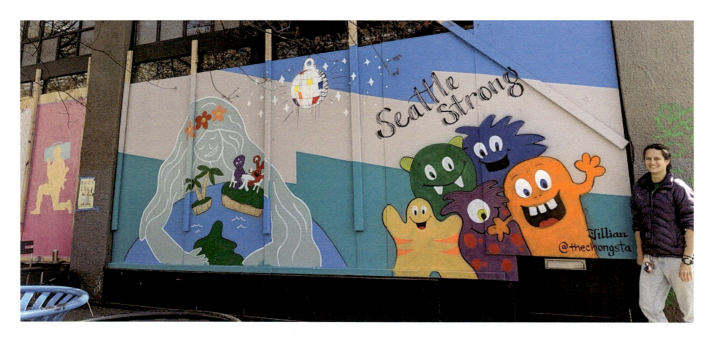

94 Photos: ARTIST

Artist:	Jillian Chong
Name of Mural:	*Make Some Noise*
Materials:	Acrylic paint, spray paint, paint markers
Size:	8 x 10 feet
Location:	Sam's Tavern, 1024 E Pike St
Artist's website:	jillianchong.com

Seattle Strong
Acrylic paint, paint markers
8 x 4 feet
Cinnaholic, 816 E Pike St
jillianchong.com

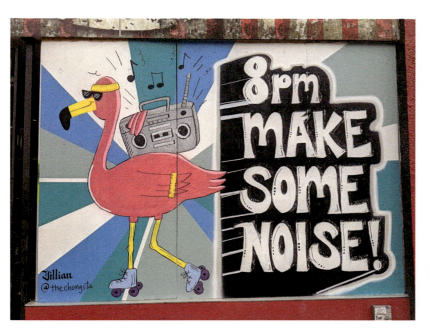 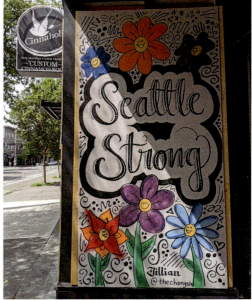

Photos: MICHELLE NEWBLOM

Artist: Jillian Chong
Name of Mural: *Don't Forget to Create*
Materials: Acrylic paint, spray paint, paint markers
Size: 6 x 18 feet
Location: Stitches, 711 E Pike St
Artist's website: jillianchong.com

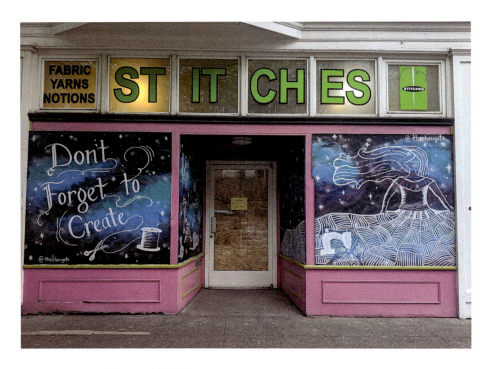

Photos: ARTIST

Artist: Josephine Rice
Crew: Kathleen Warren, Sara Pohl
Name of Mural: *PORTALdemic*
Materials: Spray paint
Size: 8 x 50 feet
Locations: Capitol Cider, 816 E Pike St
Cinnaholic, 816 E Pike St
Artist's website: josephinerice.com

"When the COVID-19 outbreak started, my work in wedding flowers went down the tubes fast. Everyone was canceling and I was out of a job. I immediately started looking for walls to paint on as murals have always been my passion. Once I did the mural at Oddfellows, the others fell into place by word of mouth. I hope my art added something pretty to the strange times."

—Josephine Rice

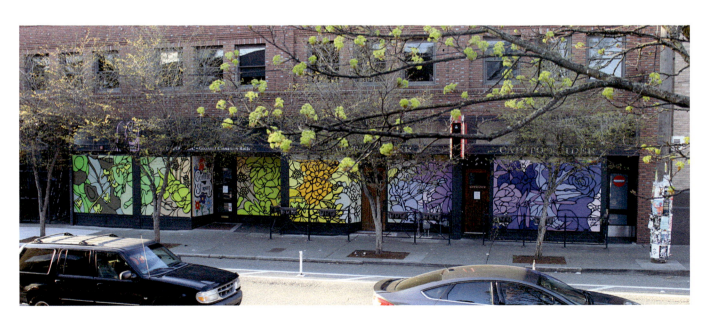

Photos: ARTIST

Artists:	Josephine Rice, Japhy Witte	
Name of Mural:	*The Serenity Prayer*	*Street Falls Quiet, Heart Does Not*
Materials:	Spray paint	Spray paint/ paint
Size:	8 x 10 feet	8 x 4 feet
Location:	Adana, 1449 E Pine St	Oddfellows, 1525 10th Ave
Coordinated by:	Shota Nakajima	josephinerice.com
Artist's website:	josephinerice.com	

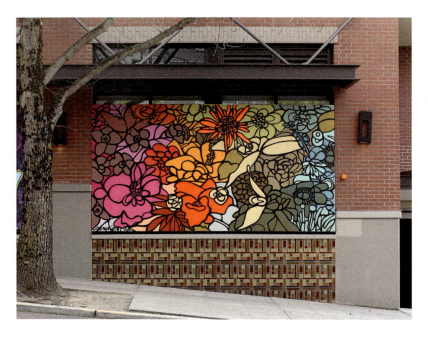
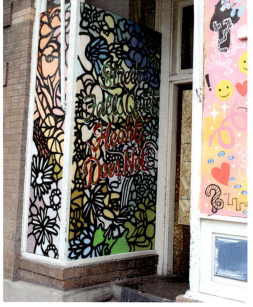

Photos: ARTIST

Artist:	SYCO
Crew:	Main, Ruby, Mosef, Naels, Atire, Guido, Sandy
Name of Mural:	*LIBERT*
Materials:	Spray paint
Size:	10 x 15 feet
Location:	QFC, 417 Broadway E
Artist's website:	@thesycopath on Instagram

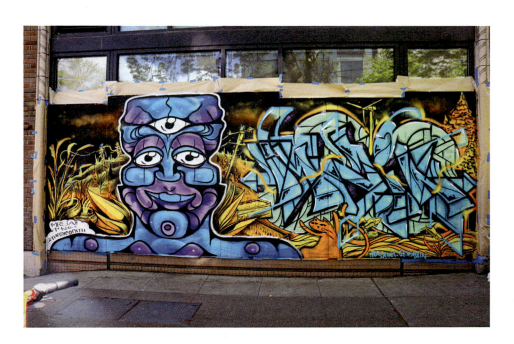

Photos: B GNARLEY

Artist:	Kalee Bly Choiniere (Barely Awake)
Name of Mural:	*Dreaming Is Part Of The Process*
Materials:	Latex paint
Size:	8 x 18 feet
Location:	Urban Outfitters, 401 Broadway E
Coordinated by:	Overall Creative
Artist's website:	barelyawakekalee.com

"Sharing art at such a large and impermanent scale gives me a moment to connect with the world in a way that feels resonant with life's unfolding."

—Kalee Bly Choiniere

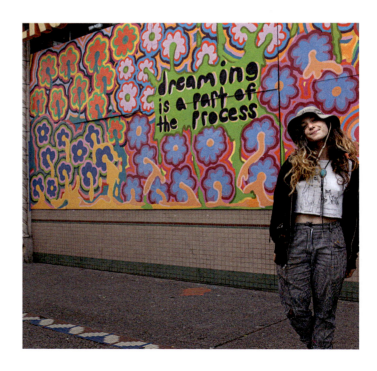

Photos: AUSTIN WILSON

Artist: Kalee Bly Choiniere (Barely Awake)
Name of Mural: *No Expectations*
Materials: Latex paint
Size: 10 x 25 feet
Location: The Baltic Room, 1207 Pine St
Artist's website: barelyawakekalee.com

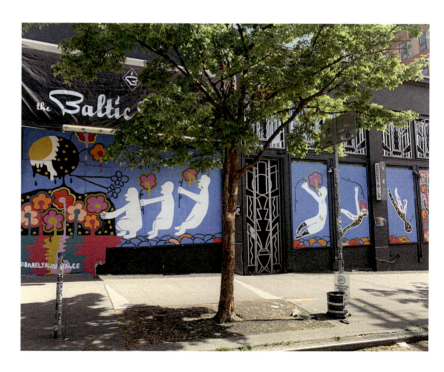

Photos: ARTIST

Artist:	Kalee Bly Choiniere (Barely Awake)	
Name of Mural:	*I Can't Wait To Dance With You*	*See You Soon*
Materials:	Latex paint	Latex paint
Size:	7 x 10 feet	15 x 20 feet
Location:	Castle Megastore, 1017 E Pike St	Quinn's Pub, 1001 E Pike St
Artist's website:	barelyawakekalee.com	barelyawakekalee.com

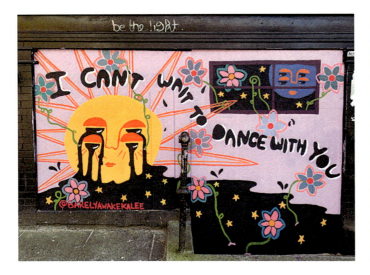 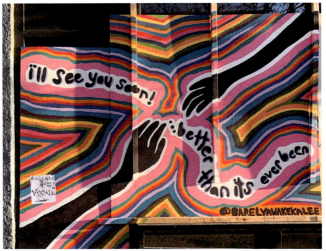

Photos: ARTIST

Artists:	Sam Trout, Kimberly Tieu
Crew:	Kathleen Warren, Lina Cholewinski, Evann Strathern
Name of Mural:	*I'll See You...When We Land*
Materials:	Paint, spray paint
Size:	8 x 92 feet
Location:	Urban Outfitters, 401 Broadway E
Coordinated by:	Overall Creative
Artist's website:	kimberlytieu.com

"As we entered into the Covid crisis I began to think a lot about how similar lock-down is to traveling in space. It's a lot of waiting in isolation, some space madness, and you'll end up on a different planet than the one you left. So saying 'I'll see you when we land,' acknowledges that dynamic and instills faith that we'll make it to the other side."

—Sam Trout

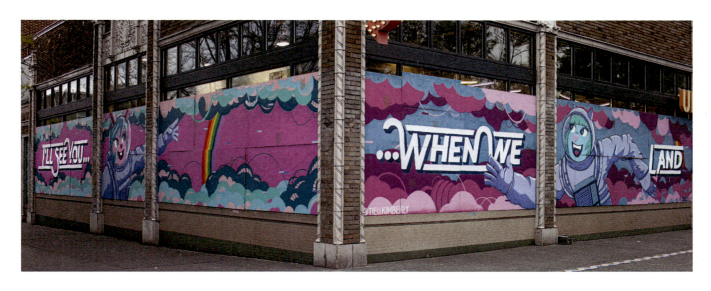

Photos: AUSTIN WILSON

Artist:	Katlyn Hubner
Name of Mural:	*Doghouse*
Materials:	Acrylic paint
Size:	8 x 25 feet
Location:	Dog House Leathers, 715 E Pike St
Artist's website:	katlynart.com

"I've always wanted to paint a mural. So when I saw all the murals going up at the beginning of quarantine, it inspired me to get involved in my local art community. I reached out to Overall Creative expressing my interest in painting a mural... and a week later, they had a wall for me! I'm so, so grateful for the opportunity the awesome OC team gave me. I had such a fun experience painting my first mural and hope it's not my last!"

—Katlyn Hubner

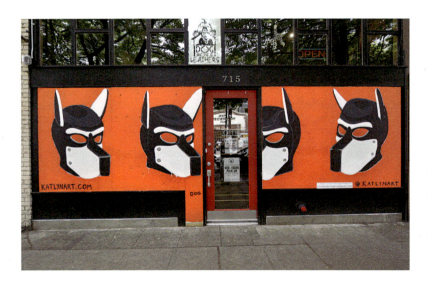 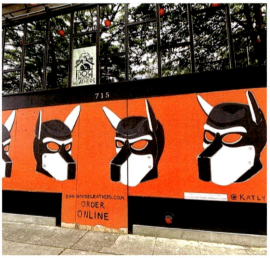

104 Photos: STEVE GILBERT

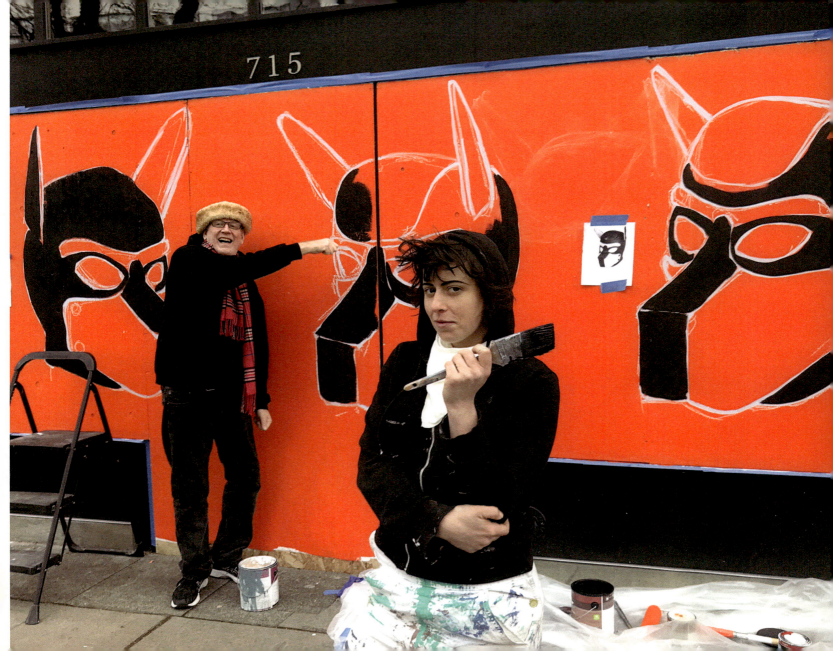

Artists:	Mari Shibuya, VK Signs
Name of Mural:	*New Systems Will Grow...*
Materials:	Exterior latex, acrylic, aerosol, love
Size:	10 x 20 feet
Location:	Le Labo, 921 E Pine St
Coordinated by:	Overall Creative
Artist's website:	marishibuya.com

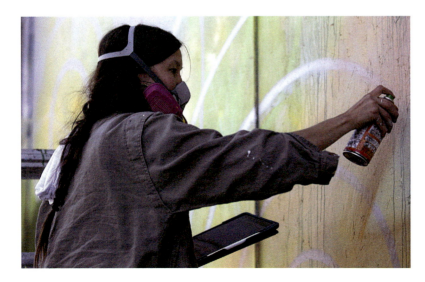

"I painted this mural because I feel it is important to put positive propaganda around us. As our world slowed down with quarantine and the onset of COVID-19, there was space to begin to imagine our world anew."

—Mari Shibuya

Photos: AUSTIN WILSON, MEGAN FARMER

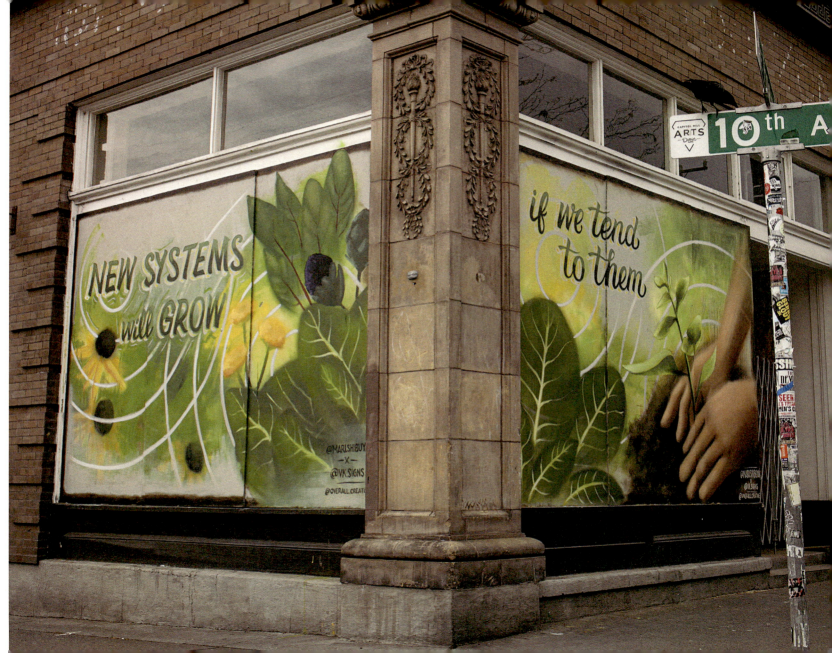

Artist:	Matt Midgley
Name of Mural:	*Untitled*
Materials:	Acrylic paint
Size:	10 x 3 feet
Location:	Urban Outfitters, 401 Broadway E
Coordinated by:	Overall Creative
Artist's website:	mattmidgley.com

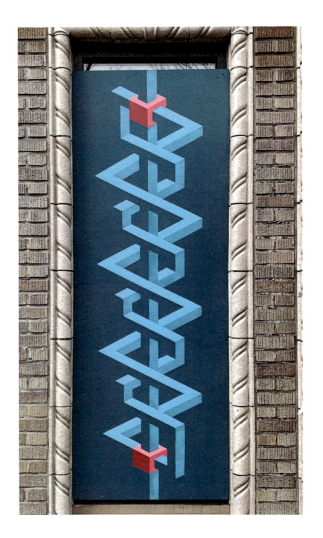

Photos: ARTIST

Artist:	Mia Pizzuto
Name of Mural:	*Bloom Where You Are Planted*
Materials:	Paint, clear varnish
Size:	9 x 8 feet
Location:	Adana Restaurant, 1449 E Pine St
Credits:	Inspired by a recent trip to the Kubota Gardens
Artist's website:	miapizzuto.com

"My hope is that this mural reminds people that we can blossom even during the darkest of times, and that we really can bloom where we are planted. Even if we are homebound and social distancing, we can still stay connected to one another and do great things. This magnolia symbolizes strength, growth and resilience—qualities we all share on this journey."

—Mia Pizzuto

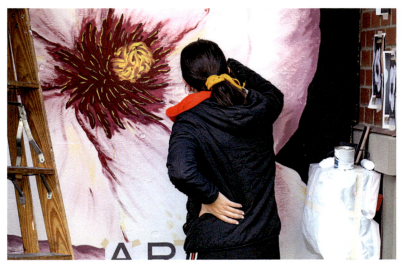
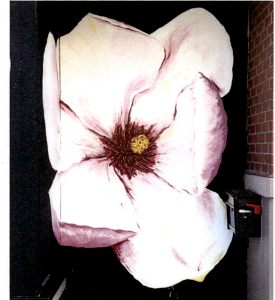

Photos: GILLIAN PECKHAM

109

Artist:	Morgan Zion
Name of Mural:	*Sam's Says, Stay Home & Keep Smiling Seattle*
Materials:	Acrylic, spray paint
Size:	9 x 50 feet
Location:	Sam's Tavern, 1024 E Pike St
Artist's website:	morganzion.co/murals

"I love to make people smile. My murals are meant to transform hopeless plywood boards and drab walls into positive, inspiring, and bright murals. Along with positive and inspiring messages, my murals contain colorful imagery representing hope, love, connection, and community. I aim to spread positivity, and brighten mindsets with every design and color I work with."

—Morgan Zion

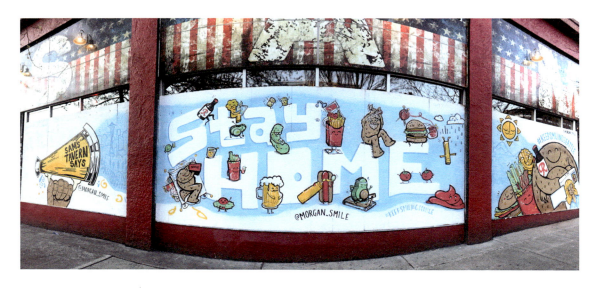

Photos: ARTIST

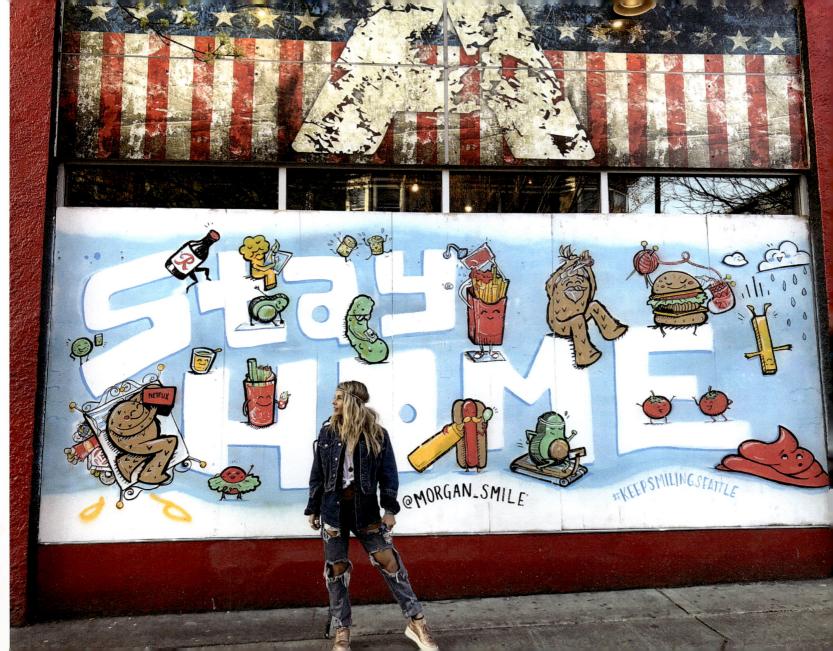

Artist: Rainbow Tay
Name of Mural: *You & I, Will Always Be Back Then*
Materials: Latex paint on plywood
Size: 8 x 16 feet
Location: Laughing Buddha Tattoo, 1534 Broadway
Coordinated by: Overall Creative
Credits: Rebecca Sugar
Artist's website: rainbowtay.com

"I wanted to share a message of hope and connectedness—to let people know that things happen and always will and that we will still be connected. Which is a message I think we all need to hear right now."

—Rainbow Tay

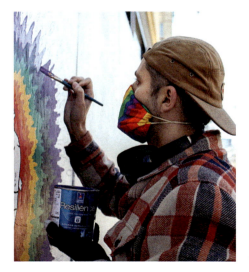
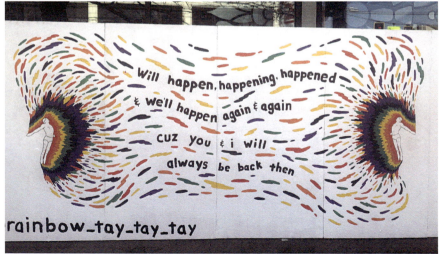

112   Photos: ARTIST, AUSTIN WILSON

Artist: Rich M. Stevens
Name of Mural: *I Can't Wait to See You Again*
Materials: Spray paint, acrylic paint
Size: 5 x 12 feet
Location: Castle Megastore, 1017 E Pike St
Coordinated by: Overall Creative
Artist's website: richmstevens.com

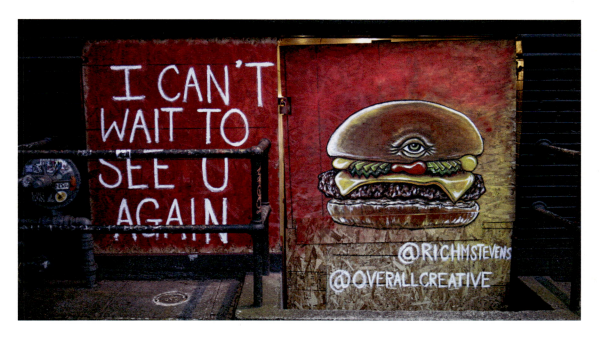

Photos: ARTIST

Artist: Ronnie Taylor
Name of Mural: *Bowie Magic*
Materials: Spray paint, acrylic
Size: 10 x 16 feet
Location: Vacant storefront, 1534 Broadway
Coordinated by: Overall Creative, Kathleen Warren
Artist's website: ronnie-art.com

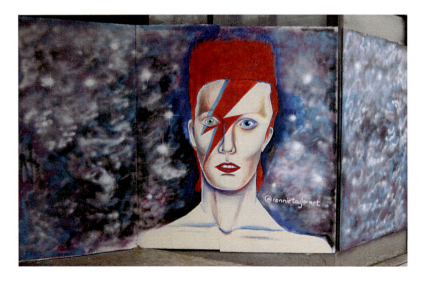

"I agreed to paint this mural of David Bowie on Broadway to celebrate the LGBT community. Since this is my first mural, I learned that while taking risks like this might seem scary, it's how you grow. Your soul stretches out into new horizons and abilities to be discovered. Not only in art, but also in life."

—Ronnie Taylor

Photos: ARTIST, AUSTIN WILSON

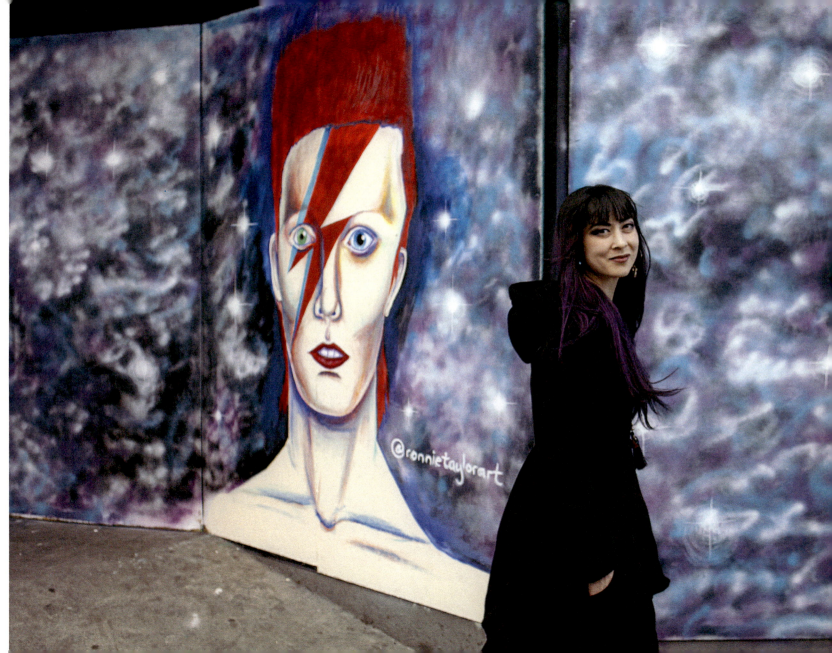

Artist: Sandy
Name of Mural: *Sandy's Pick n' Pull*
Materials: Belton Premium on latex
Size: 5 x 11 feet
Location: Chase Bank, 1429 Broadway
Coordinated by: Overall Creative
Artist's website: @paint_2_change on Instagram

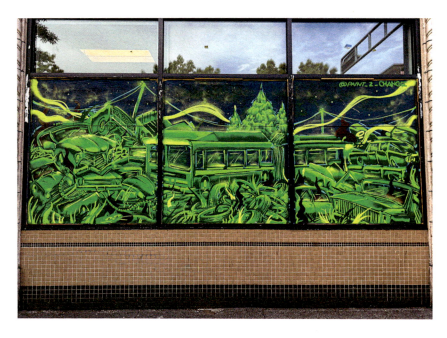

Photos: MATTHEW MACDONALD

Artist: Sandy
Name of Mural: *Late Night Freakout*
Materials: Rustoleum on latex
Size: 9 x 15 feet
Location: Capitol Coffee Works, 907 E Pike Street
Coordinated by: Morgan
Artist's website: @paint_2_change on Instagram

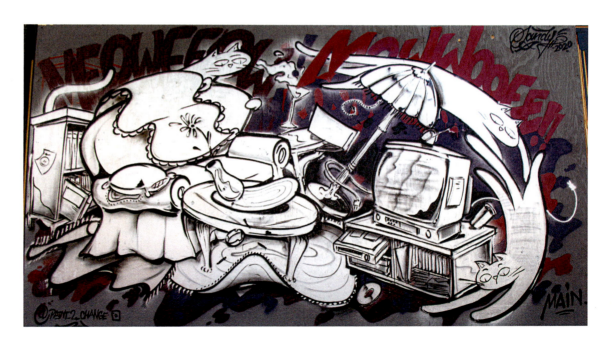

Photos: MATTHEW MACDONALD

Artist:	Sandy
Crew:	Bailee Hiatt
Name of Mural:	*Doubled-Down Dogs*
Materials:	Mixed latex, enamel
Size:	8 x 15 feet
Location:	8oz Burger, 1401 Broadway
Artist's website:	@paint_2_change on Instagram

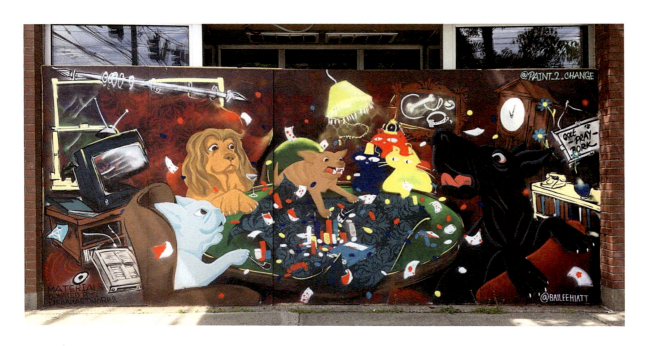

Photos: MATTHEW MACDONALD

Artists: Tara Velan, Sandy
Name of Mural: *Support WANMA*
Materials: Exterior paint, spray paint
Size: 8 x 36 feet
Location: Neumos, 925 E Pike St
Coordinated by: Washington Nightlife Music Association
Artist's website: @yesitstara on Instagram

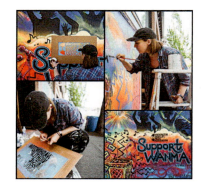

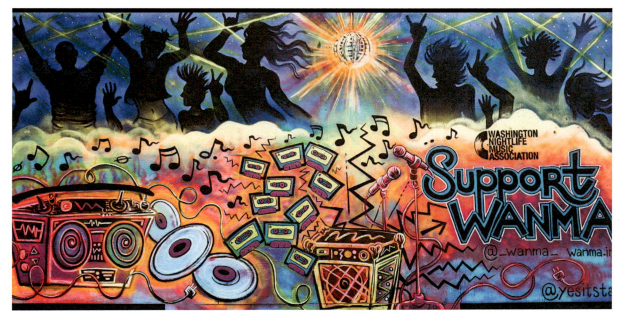

Photos: JAKE GRAVBROT

Artist: Shogo Ota
Name of Mural: *We Got This*
Materials: Spray paint (stencil), acrylic (brush)
Size: 6 x 8 feet
Location: Adana, 1449 E Pine St
Coordinated by: Shota Nakajima
Artist's website: tiremanstudio.com

"This was something I could do to use to use my skills to support the community and spread some good vibes!"

—Shogo Ota

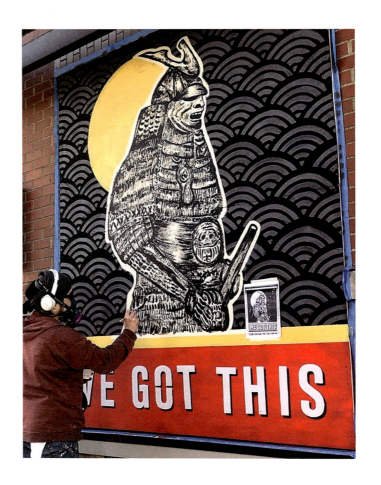

120 Photos: ARTIST, SHOTA NAKAJIMA

Artist:	Tara Velan	
Name of Mural:	*Strength*	*You Are Essential!*
Materials:	Exterior paint	Exterior paint
Size:	6 x 8 feet	4 x 8 feet
Location:	Wildrose Bar, 1021 E Pike St	Castle Megastore, 1017 E Pike St
Coordinated by:	Katie Conover	Katie Conover
Artist's website:	@yesitstara on Instagram	

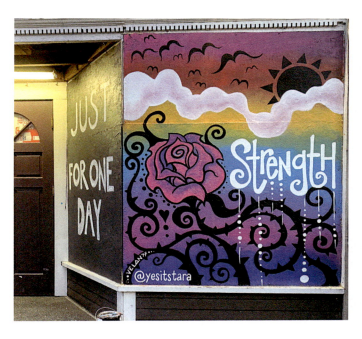
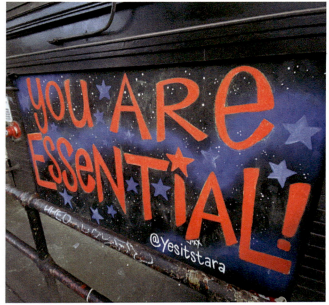

Photos: ARTIST

121

Artist:	They Drift
Crew:	Ksra
Name of Mural:	*Stay Healthy*
Materials:	Spray paint
Size:	8 x 36 feet
Location:	Broadway and East 901 E Pike St
Artist's website:	@ksra_ksra on Instagram
	@theydrift on Instagram

"My wife Ksra and I were inspired by what's going on in the world. We wanted to let everyone know that staying home is the best way to stay safe, though not always an option, and that if you have to go out, please protect yourself to stay healthy."

—They Drift

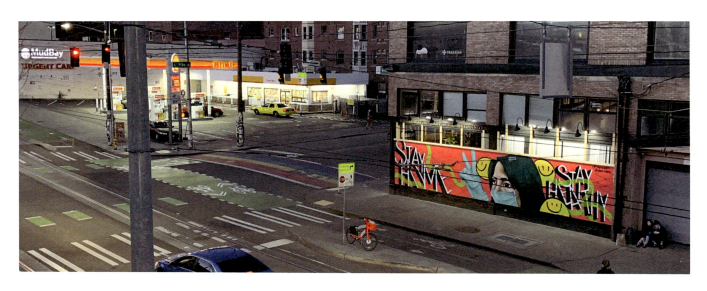

Photos: ARTIST

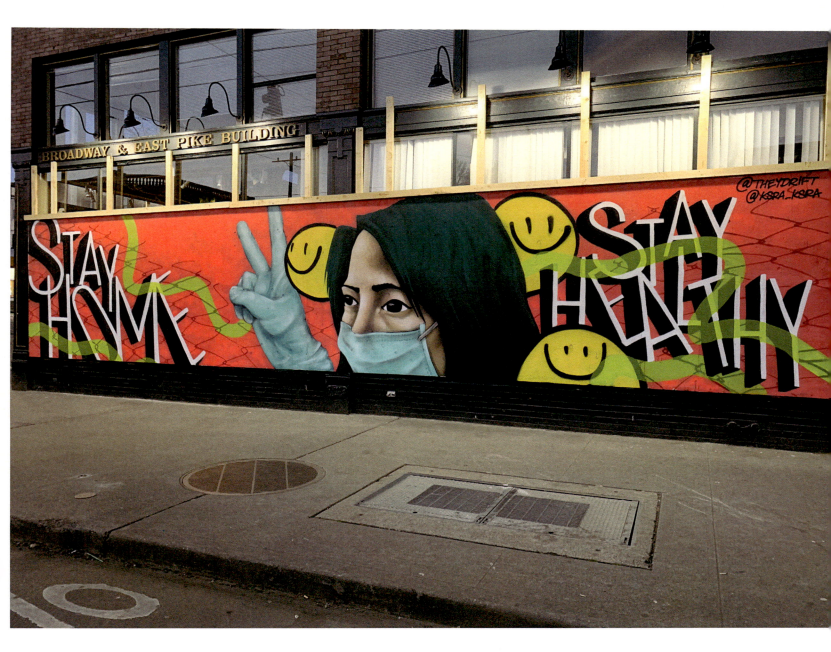

Artist:	Will Schlough
Name of Mural:	*Untitled*
Materials:	Acrylic on ACX plywood cutouts
Size:	8 x 8 feet
Location:	The Runaway, 1425 10th Ave
Coordinated by:	Overall Creative
Artist's website:	willschlough.com

"I'm always amazed by just how much art can accomplish. In times of uncertainty, we long for a feeling of togetherness. Art can step in to help bridge the gap between us in times of uncertainty and separation. Beyond an opportunity to make work for the public to enjoy, this project was a unique chance to join forces with a community of talented artists, even if it was from a distance."

—Will Schlough

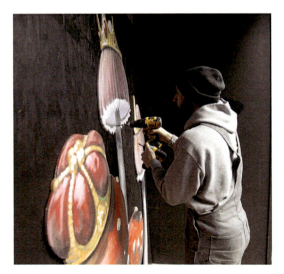 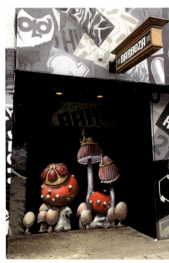 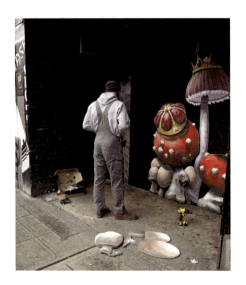

Photos: ARTIST, LINDSAY THOMAS

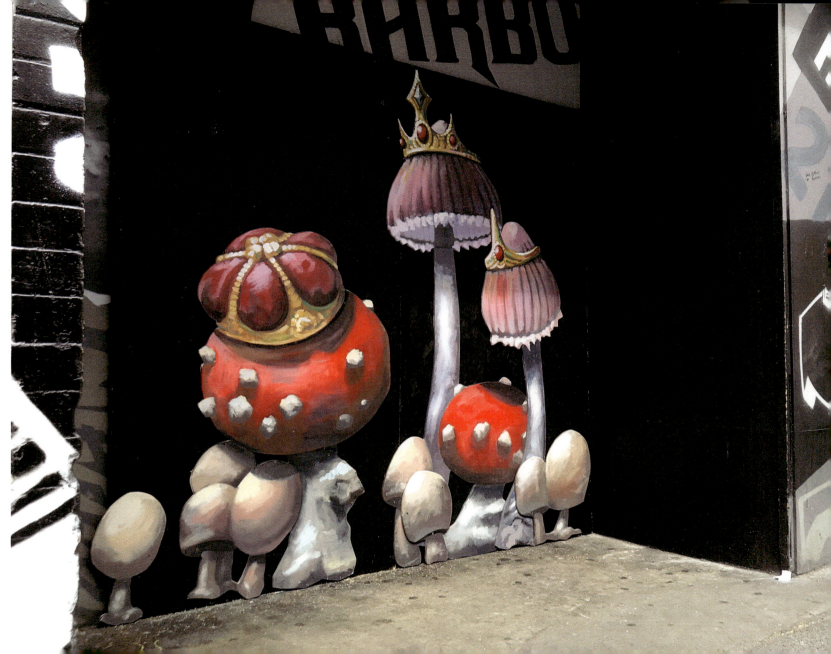

Artist: Zach Rockstad
Crew: Marry Tonnu
Name of Mural: *John Prine Ridin' the Main Line*
Materials: Mixed Media (aerosol, acrylic, solid marker)
Size: 8 x 20 feet
Location: Life on Mars, 722 E Pike St
Coordinated by: Overall Creative
Credits: John Prine (text of quote)
Artist's website: zachrockstad.com

"I painted the mural because I wanted to donate my stagnant time to making art and filling up these boarded-up, blank spaces. I was offered and commissioned this piece about musician John Prine, who was taken by the coronavirus, to honor him and serve as a reminder that you are not alone during these very isolating and confusing times."

—Zach Rockstad

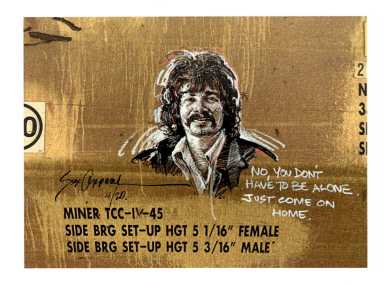

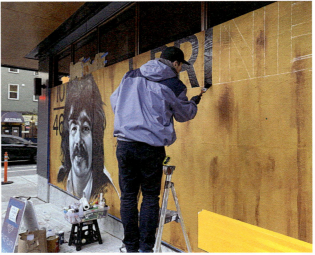

Photos: ARTIST

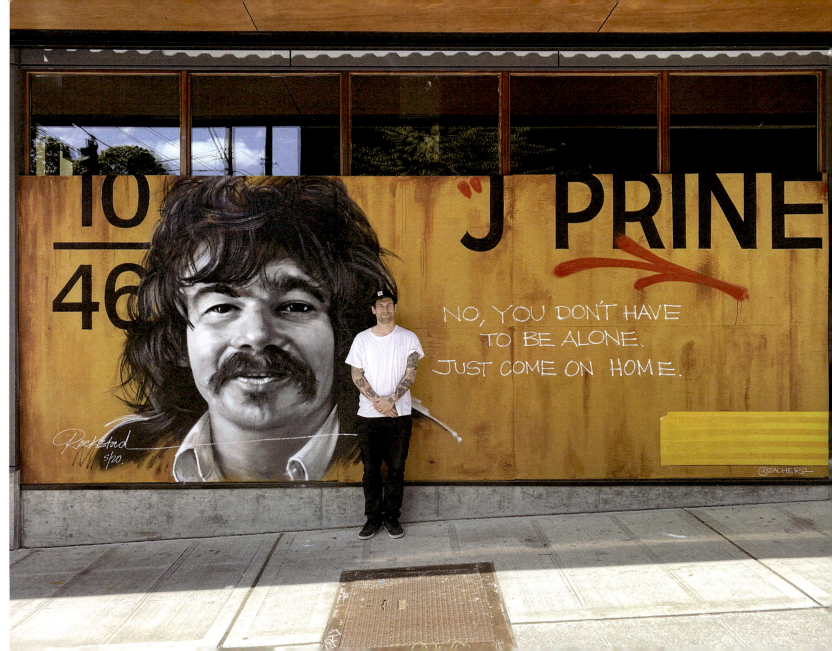

Artist: Zaeos
Name of Mural: *Orange Bloom*
Materials: Latex, spray paint
Size: 7 x 24 feet
Location: The Runaway, 1425 10th Ave
Coordinated by: Overall Creative, Linda Derschang Group, CES Studio
Artist's website: @zaeos on Instagram

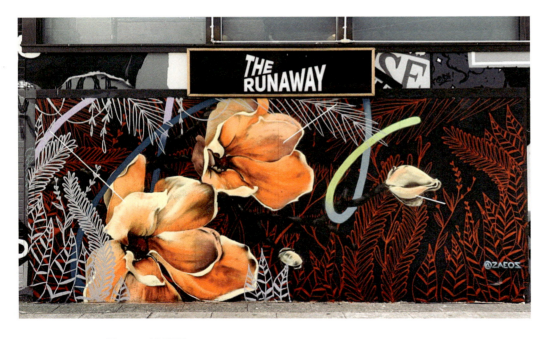

Photos: ARTIST

Artist:	Zaeos	
Name of Mural:	*Gray Floral*	*Corvid*
Materials:	Latex, spray paint	Latex, spray paint
Size:	5 x 6 feet	8 x 6 feet
Location:	Linda's, 707 E Pine St	CES Studio, 1428 10th Ave
Coordinated by:	Overall Creative, Linda Derschang Group, CES Studio	Overall Creative, Linda Derschang Group, CES Studio
Artist's website:	@zaeos on Instagram	

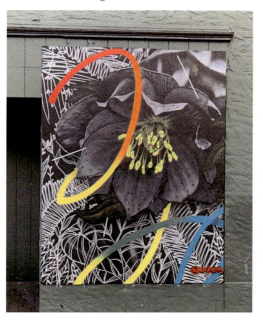
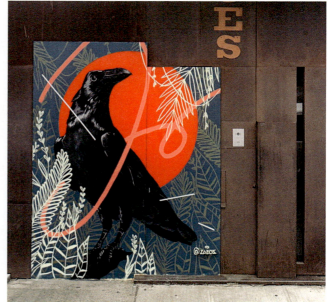

Photos: ARTIST

Artist:	Kreau
Name of Mural:	*We'll Find a Way*
Materials:	Spray acrylic on plywood, stencil
Size:	7 x 8 feet
Location:	Honor Coffee, 131 Broadway E
Artist's website:	kreau.com

"For better or worse, Seattle is a city of growth. It has life behind every wall and window. To see that life suddenly boarded up is a powerful and profound experience. Seattle also used to have a lot more murals. However, many of those have started to disappear from our streets.

On one hand, our architecture has changed— buildings are tall glass towers with little room for large pieces of art. On the other hand, the same growth that gives Seattle life has also presented many challenges for certain communities, including the artist community. A lot of the vibrant arts spaces of many years ago have been pushed further out of the city or have been spread thin due to gentrification. Murals themselves have started to become indoor fixtures in offices rather than public pieces.

It has all been a bit disheartening. Yet when I grabbed some stencils and a few cans, I suddenly saw the artist community rallying behind a common goal. Because of COVID-19, that dispersed group has found a common place again: the streets. Boarded-up businesses afforded us a bittersweet opportunity to spread messages of hope, empathy, joy, frustration, or whatever else needed to be said."

—Kreau

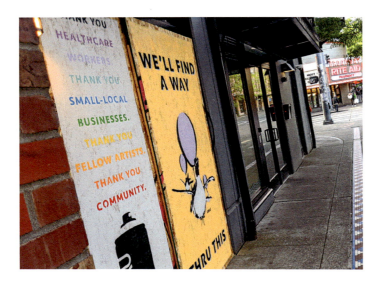

Photos: ARTIST

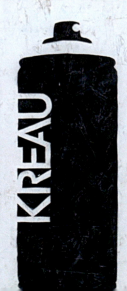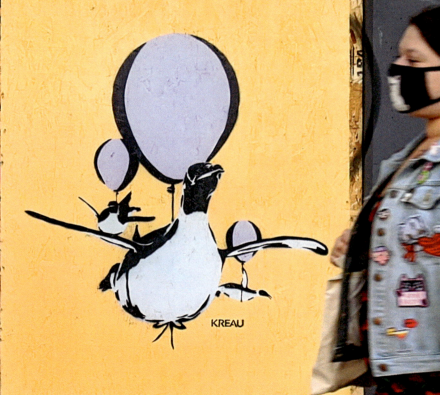

Artist: Kreau
Name of Mural: *Make a Joyful Noise*
Materials: Spray acrylic on plywood, stencil
Size: 8 x 8 feet
Location: Quinn's Pub, 1001 E Pike St
Artist's website: kreau.com

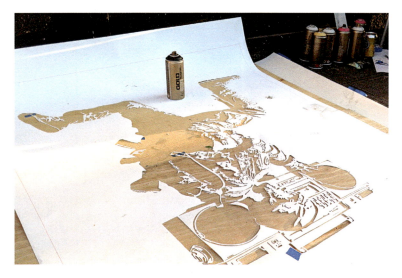
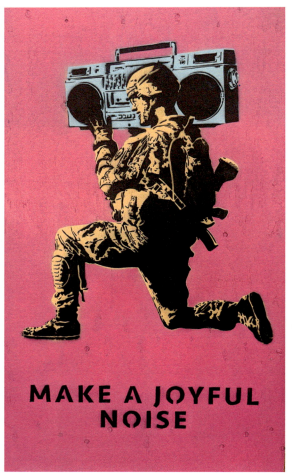

Photos: ARTIST

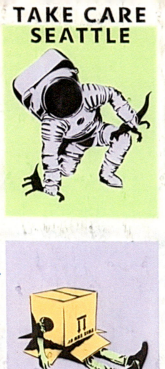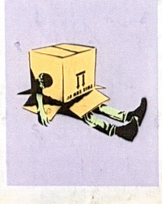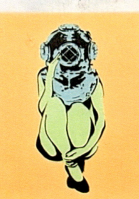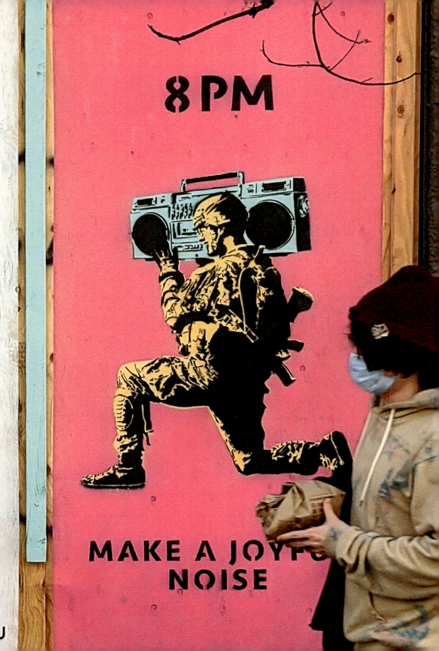

Artist:	Kreau	
Name of Mural:	*Safety Is Sexy*	*Imagination Not Isolation*
Materials:	Spray acrylic on plywood, stencil	Spray acrylic on plywood, stencil
Size:	2 x 6 feet	6 x 5.5 feet
Location:	The Doctor's Office, 1631 E Olive Way	Saint John's, 719 E Pike
Coordinated by:	Dozfy	
Artist's website:	kreau.com	

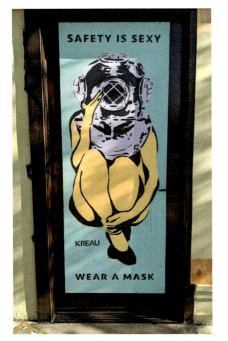
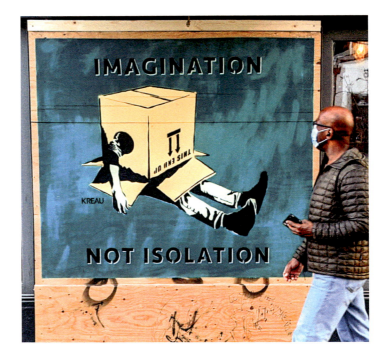

Photos: ARTIST

First Hill

Artists:	Jillian Chong, Gretchen Proulx
Name of Mural:	*Together We Will Rise*
Materials:	Acrylic paint, spray paint, acrylic markers
Size:	8 x 42.5 feet
Location:	Copymart, 1018 Seneca St
Artist's website:	jillianchong.com

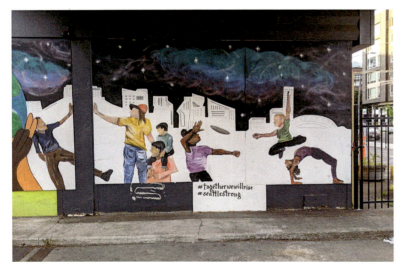

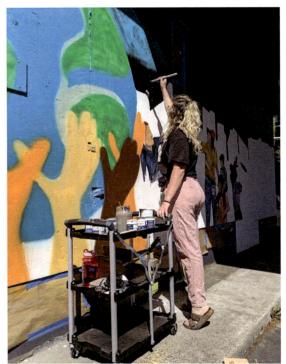

Photos: ARTIST

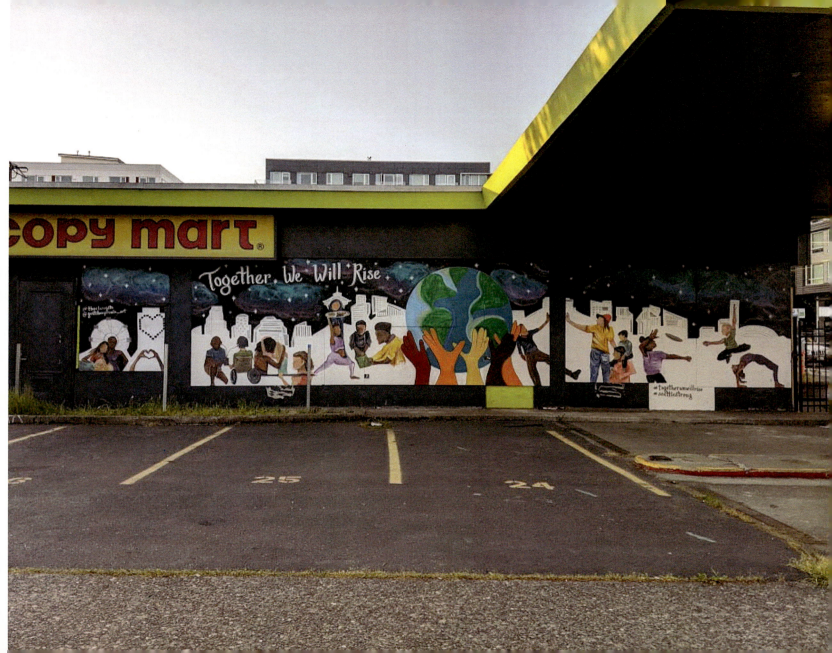

International District
SODO

Artist: Sandy
Name of Mural: *Sandy's Scrapyard*
Materials: Rustoleum on latex
Size: 8 x 16 feet
Location: Saeteun's Garage, 720 S Jackson St
Coordinated by: Saeteun
Artist's website: @paint_2_change on Instagram

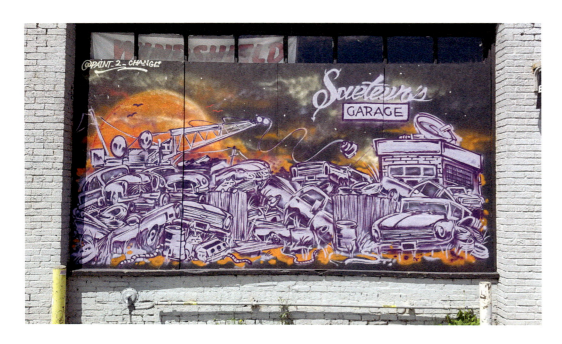

Photos: B. GNARLY

Artist: Antonio Varchetta
Name of Mural: *Peaceful Encounter*
Materials: Spray paint on plywood
Size: 20 x 7 feet
Location: Chu Minh, 12th and Jackson
Coordinated by: @antonio.sprays on Instagram

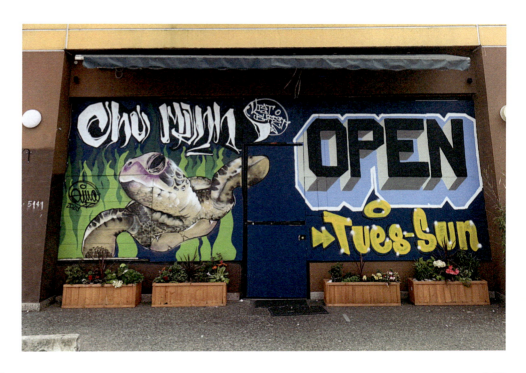

Photos: ARTIST

Artist: Ariel Parrow
Name of Mural: *Untitled*
Materials: Acrylic paint
Size: 9 x 20 feet
Location: National Corporate Housing, 2444 1st Ave S
Coordinated by: Lauren Ross
Artist's website: thechaoticaquatic.com

"Kathleen Warren (of Overall Creative) reached out and asked if I had any interest in painting and I absolutely did! Sunsets and the sky are so soothing, and it felt like the right time to paint something that would give people a sense of peace and calm."

—Ariel Parrow

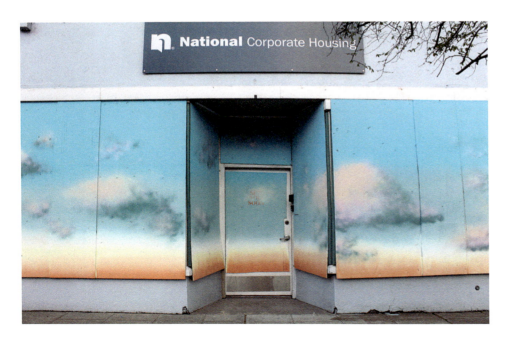

142 Photos: ARTIST

Artist: Lina Cholewinski
Name of Mural: *See You Later, Alligator*
Materials: Acrylic latex
Size: 10 x 30 feet
Location: Rejuvenation, 2910 1st Ave S
Coordinated by: Lauren Ross
Artist's website: @bonesandgold on Instagram

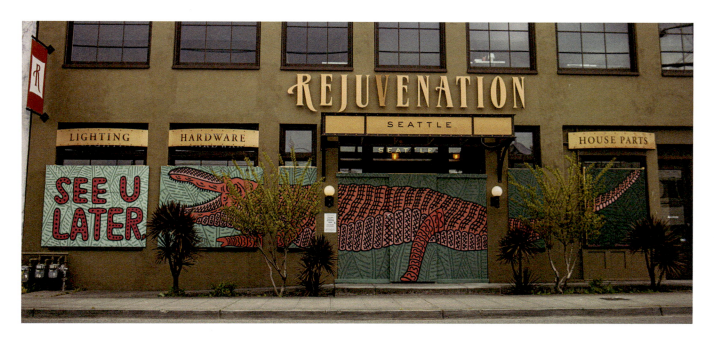

Photos: LAUREN ROSS

Artist: LillyBomb
Name of Mural: *Golden Rule*
Materials: Aerosol, house paint
Size: 8 x 6 feet
Location: Hawks Nest, 1028 1st Ave S
Coordinated by: Kathleen Warren at Overall Creative
Artist's website: Chriskentart.com

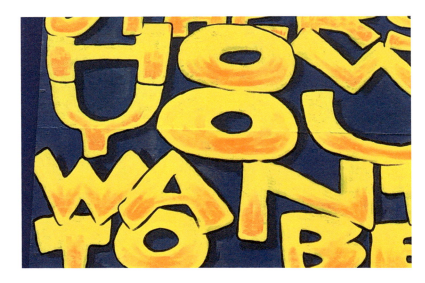

"With everything going on, I wanted to say something simple that everyone could get behind."

—LillyBomb

Photos: CHRIS KENT

TREAT OTHERS YOU WANT TO BE TREATED

©LILLY_B_0_M_B

Artist: Reed Olsen
Name of Mural: *Show Up*
Materials: Acrylic paint
Size: 9 x 4 feet
Location: Hawks Nest, 1028 1st Ave
Coordinated by: Overall Creative
Artist's website: reedonwheels.net

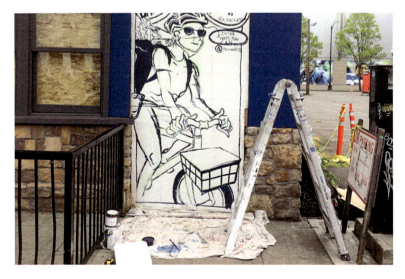
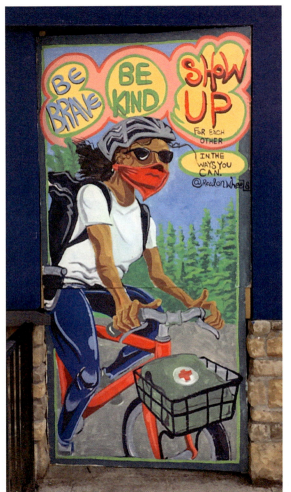

Photos: ARTIST

Queen Anne

Artist:	Andrew Miller
Name of Mural:	*Queen Anne Loves You*
Materials:	Acrylic house paint
Size:	4 x 24 feet
Location:	Targy's Tavern, 600 W Crockett St.
Coordinated by:	Targy's Tavern, Joel Stedman
Artist's website:	mantisart.com

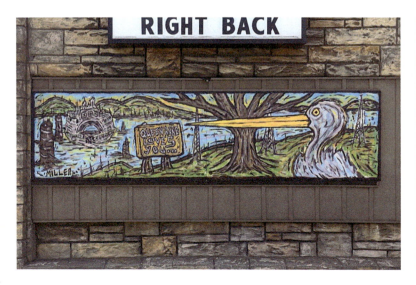
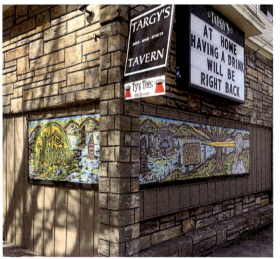

Photos: ARTIST

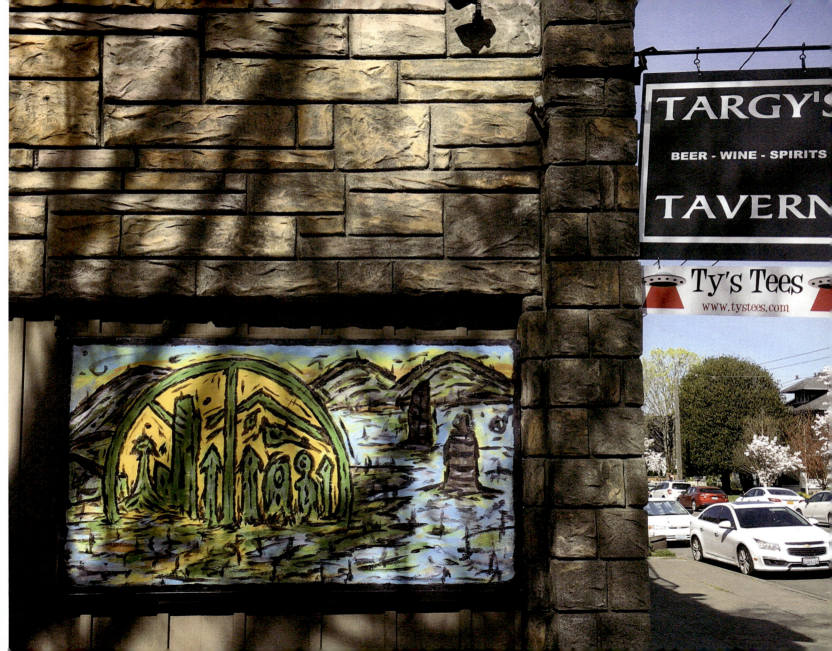

Artist: Andrew Miller
Name of Mural: *Out and Under at Sea*
Materials: Acrylic house paint
Size: 8 x 84 feet
Location: Lee Properties, 6th Ave W and W Crockett
Coordinated by: Beverly Hunnicutt
Artist's website: mantisart.com

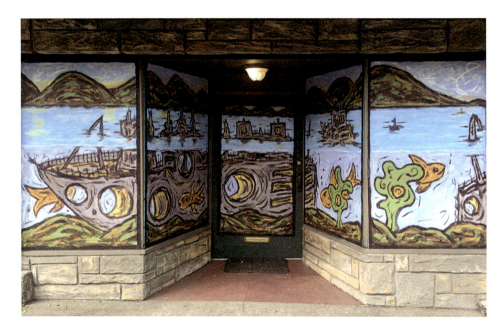

150   Photos: ARTIST

Artist: Antonio Varchetta
Name of Mural: *Untitled*
Materials: Spray paint
Size: 10 x 7 feet
Location: Big Mario's, 815 5th Ave N
Coordinated by: Devin Reynolds
Credits: Art Primo
Artist's website: @antonio.sprays on Instagram

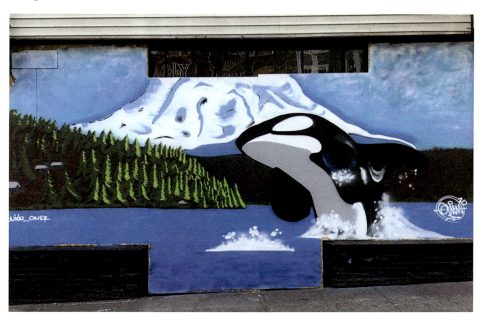

Photos: ARTIST

Artist: Burgandy Viscosi
Name of Mural: *Healthy Lungs*
Materials: Acrylic
Size: 4 x 9 feet
Location: Counterbalance Barber Shop, 1424 Queen Anne N
Artist's website: burgandyviscosi.com

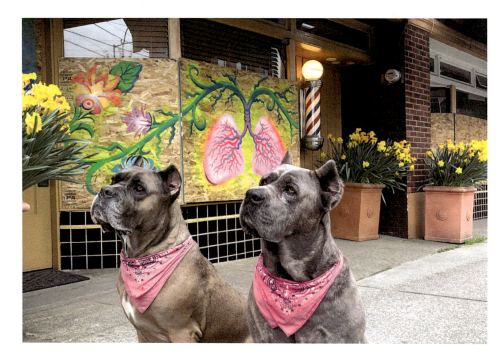

Photos: MALIA HUNTER

Artist:	Dozfy
Name of Mural:	*Stay Strong*
Materials:	Latex, oil, acrylic paint
Size:	2.5 x 5 feet
Location:	Bite Box, 307 W McGraw St
Coordinated by:	Sharon Fillingim
Artist's website:	Dozfy.net

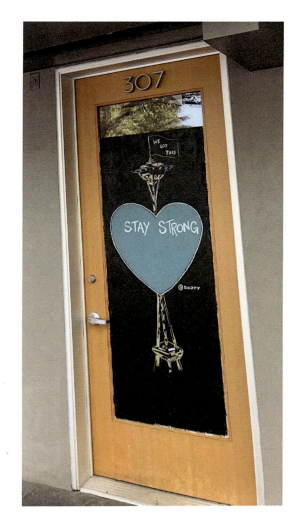

Photos: ARTIST

Fremont

Artist: Sandy
Name of Mural: *Salsa Con Sandy*
Materials: Belton spray paint on latex
Size: 9 x 11 feet
Location: Salsa Con Todo, 211 N 36th St
Artist's website: @paint_2_change on Instagram

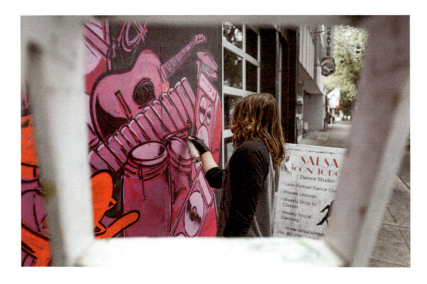

Photos: JAKE G.

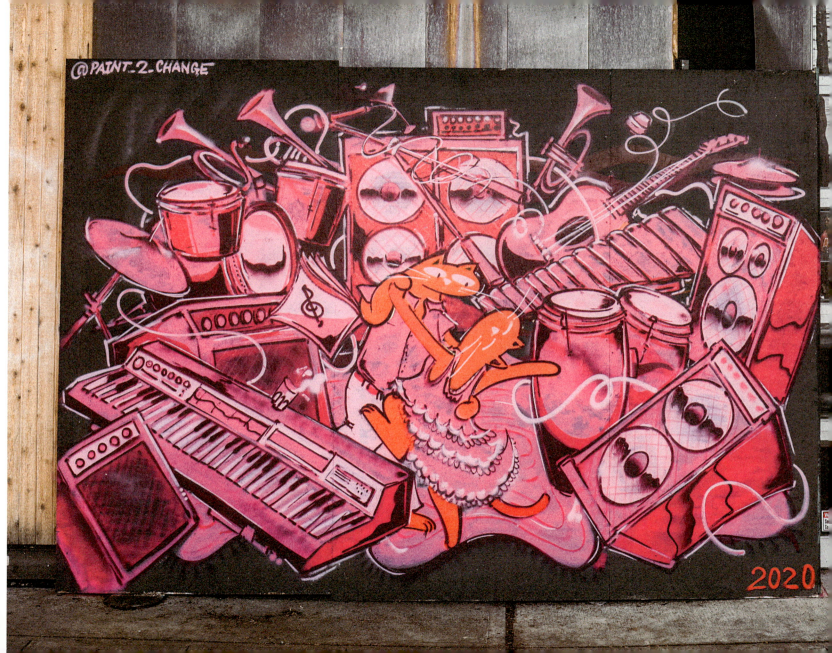

Artist: Sandy
Name of Mural: *Sandy's Hobbyshop*
Materials: Rustoleum on latex
Size: 4 x 9 feet
Location: George and Dragon, 206 N 36th St
Artist's website: @paint_2_change on Instagram

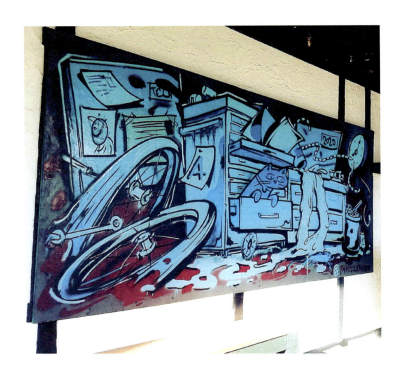

Photos: MATTHEW MACDONALD

Artist: Sandy, Bailee Hiatt
Name of Mural: *Clout King*
Materials: Latex and Rustoleum
Size: 10 x 22 feet
Location: Rudy's Barbershop, 475 N 36th St
Artist's website: @baileehiatt on Instagram

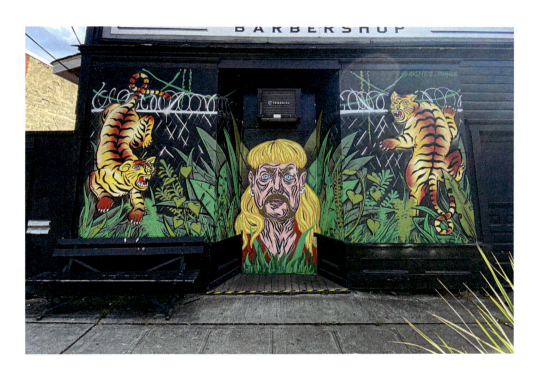

Photos: MATTHEW MACDONALD

Artist: Tara Velan
Name of Mural: *Magician's Jaybird*
Materials: Acrylic paint
Size: 4 x 12 feet
Location: Esters Enoteca, 3416 Fremont Ave N
Coordinated by: Nick and Trish Carlino
Artist's website: @yesitstara on Instagram

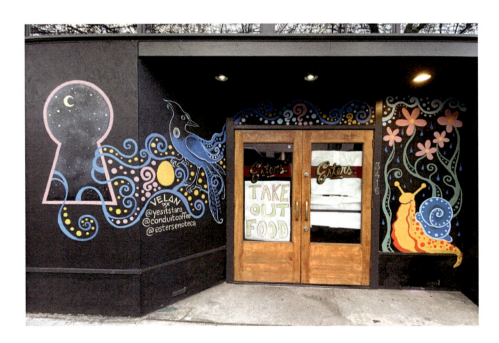

Photos: ARTIST

Ballard

Artist: Andrew Miller
Name of Mural: *The Essential Ballard Loves You*
Materials: Acrylic house paint
Size: 5 x 40 feet
Location: The Market Arms, 2401 NW Market St
Coordinated by: Ballard Alliance
Artist's website: mantisart.com

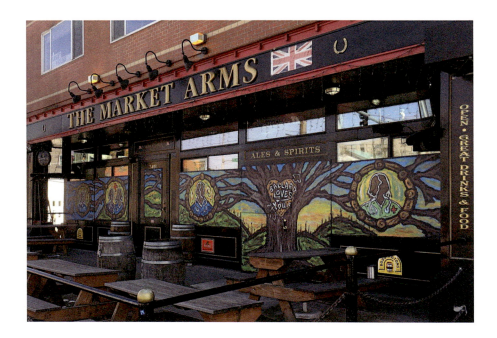

Photos: ARTIST

Artist: Andrew Miller
Name of Mural: *London Calling from the Tractor*
Materials: Acrylic house paint
Size: 8 x 18 feet
Location: Tractor Tavern, 5213 Ballard Ave NW
Coordinated by: Ballard Alliance
Artist's website: mantisart.com

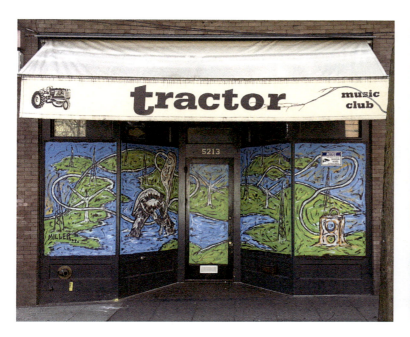 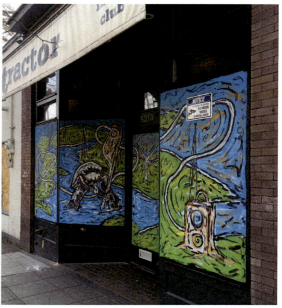

Photos: ARTIST

Artist:	Andrew Miller
Name of Mural:	*Slainte Maith - Good Health*
Materials:	Acrylic house paint
Size:	8 x 20 feet
Location:	Conor Byrne Pub, 5140 Ballard Ave
Coordinated by:	Conor Byrne Pub, Ballard Alliance
Artist's website:	mantisart.com

Real. Old. Ballard...
Acrylic house paint
4 x 16 feet
Sloop Tavern, 2830 NW Market St
Much love to Mr. Patrick Files...

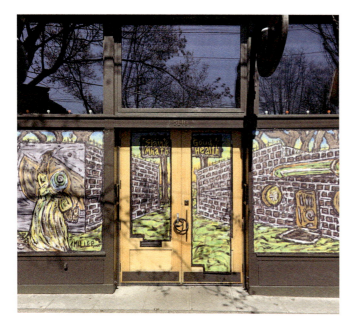 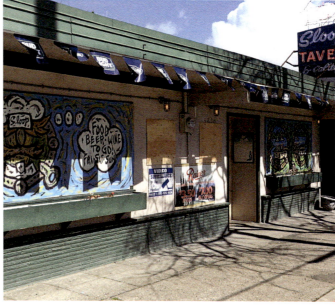

Photos: ARTIST

Artist:	Andrew Miller	
Name of Mural:	*The Hummingbird Knows...*	*All the Essentials*
Materials:	Acrylic house paint	Acrylic house paint
Size:	4 x 32 feet	4 x 60 feet
Location:	Ballard Annex, 5410 Ballard Ave NW	Vacant Storefront, 3901 Leary Way NW
Coordinated by:	Ballard Alliance	Michael Lee, Lee Properties
Artist's website:	mantisart.com	

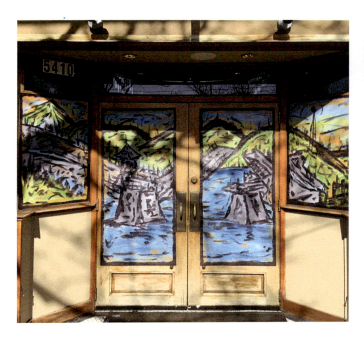 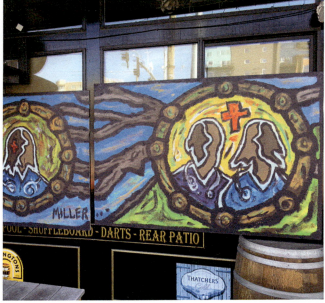

Photos: ARTIST

Artist:	Bekah Malover
Name of Mural:	*Mouthy*
Materials:	Paint
Size:	10 x 20 feet
Location:	Kathy Casey Food Studio, 5130 Ballard Ave NW
Coordinated by:	Devin Reynolds with Ballard Alliance
Artist's website:	bekahmalover.com

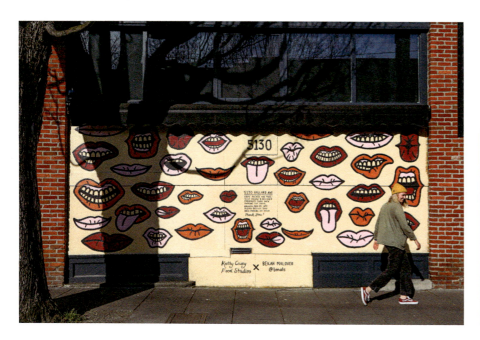

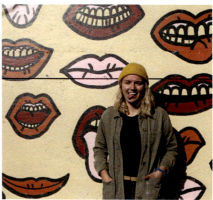

Photos: TANNA SOLBERG

Artist:	Bekah Malover
Name of Mural:	*Untitled*
Materials:	Paint
Size:	7 x 20 feet
Location:	Rudy's Barbershop, 5229 Ballard Ave NW
Coordinated by:	Devin Reynolds with Ballard Alliance
Credits:	Ballard Alliancd, Novo Painting
Artist's website:	bekahmalover.com

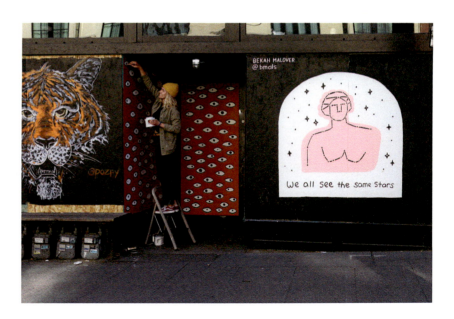

Photos: TANNA SOLBERG

Artist: Antonio Varchetta
Name of Mural: *Untitled*
Materials: Spray paint
Size: 6 x 30 feet
Location: Patagonia, 5443 Ballard Ave NW
Coordinated by: Devin Reynolds
Credits: Art Primo
Artist's website: @antonio.sprays on Instagram

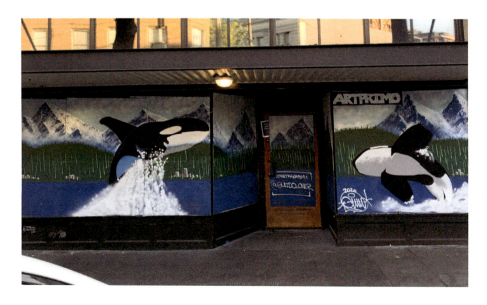

Photos: ARTIST

Artist:	Dozfy
Name of Mural:	*Untitled*
Materials:	Paint (acrylic and latex)
Size:	10 x 10 feet
Location:	Rudy's, 5229 Ballard Avenue NW
Coordinated by:	Devin Reynolds
Artist's website:	dozfy.net

Untitled
Latex, acrylic paint
4 x 5 feet each
Mean Sandwich, 1510 NW Leary Way

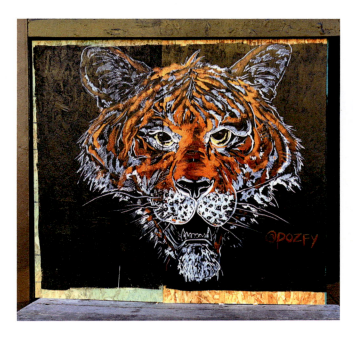
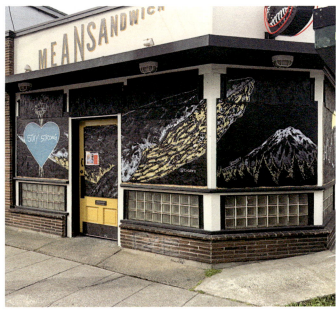

Photos: ARTIST

Artist:	Dozfy
Name of Mural:	*Untitled*
Materials:	Paint (latex, acrylic, enamel)
Size:	Four 8 x 10 foot panels
Location:	Lucca's Great Finds, 5332 Ballard Ave NW
Coordinated by:	Devin Reynolds
Artist's website:	dozfy.net

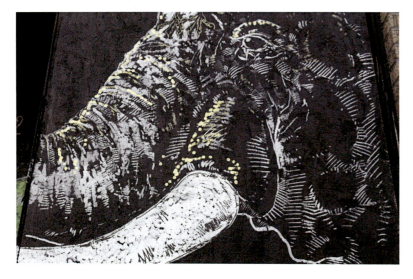
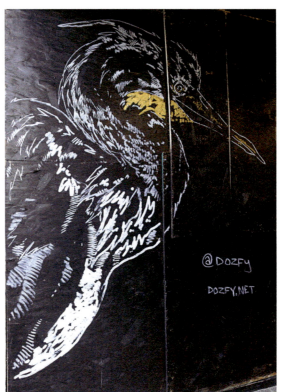

Photos: ARTIST

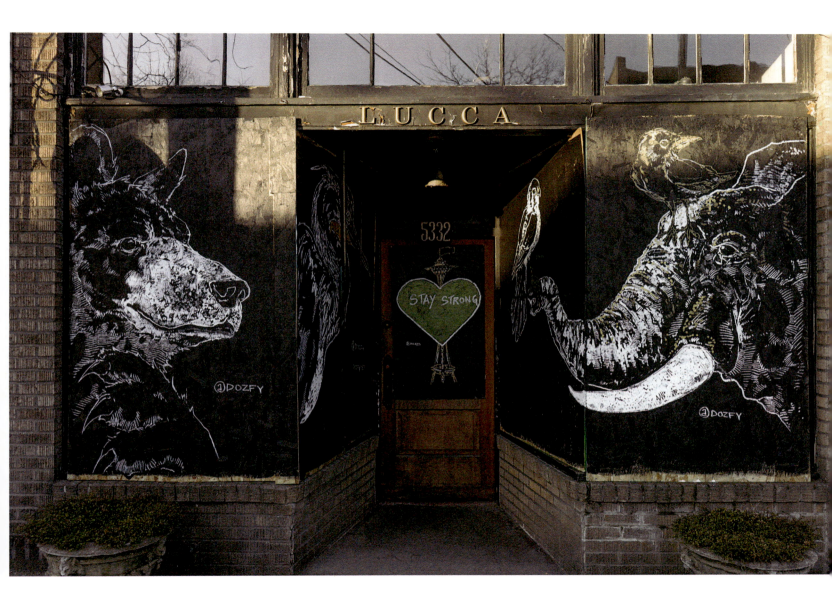

Artists:	Dozfy	
Name of Mural:	*Stay Strong*	*King's Crown*
Materials:	Latex, oil, acrylic paint	Latex, acrylic paint
Size:	3 x 4 feet	4 x 4 feet
Location:	Shingletown Saloon, 2016 NW Market St	King's Hardware, 5225 Ballard Avenue NW
Coordinated by:	Shingletown Saloon	Linda Derschang
Artist's website:	dozfy.net	

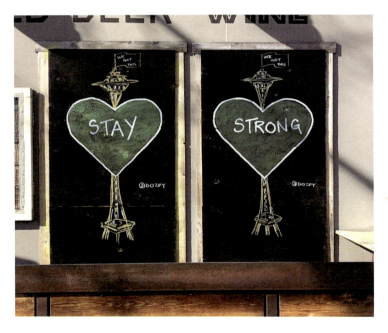 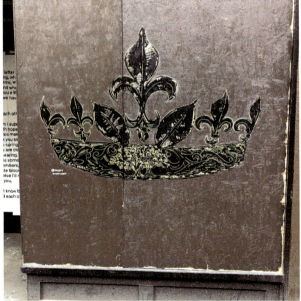

172   Photos: ARTIST

Artist: Josephine Rice
Name of Mural: *Enjoy the Flowers*
Materials: Spray paint
Size: 6 x 30 feet
Location: Venue Ballard, 5408 22nd Ave NW
Artist's website: josephinerice.com

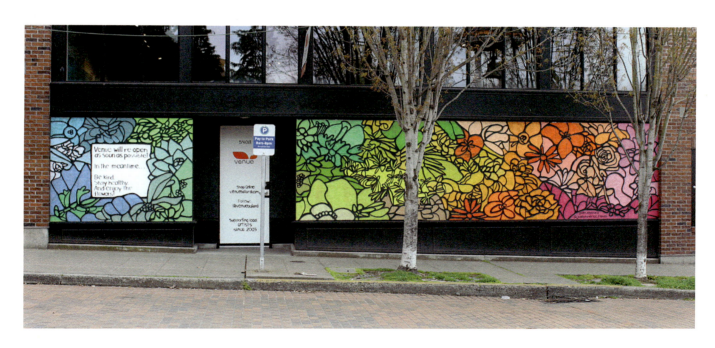

Photos: HAL PETERSON

Artist: Glynn Rosenberg
Name of Mural: *Until Next Time*
Materials: Aerosol, latex paint
Size: 8 x 15 feet
Location: Kathy Casey Food Studios, 5130 Ballard Ave NW
Coordinated by: Visit Ballard, Devin Reynolds
Artist's website: glynn35.wixsite.com/glynnrosenberg

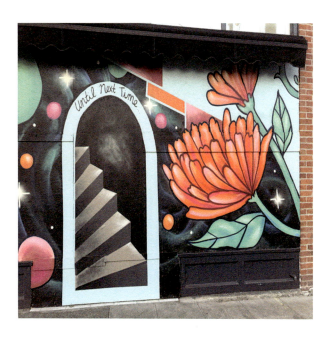

"I got involved in the project because I wanted to support my community during the pandemic, a crisis that further intensified the divide between the rich and poor. Street art can bring art to those who otherwise may not be able to experience it. With venues and galleries closed, access to art has a whole new meaning."

—Glynn Rosenberg

Photos: ARTIST

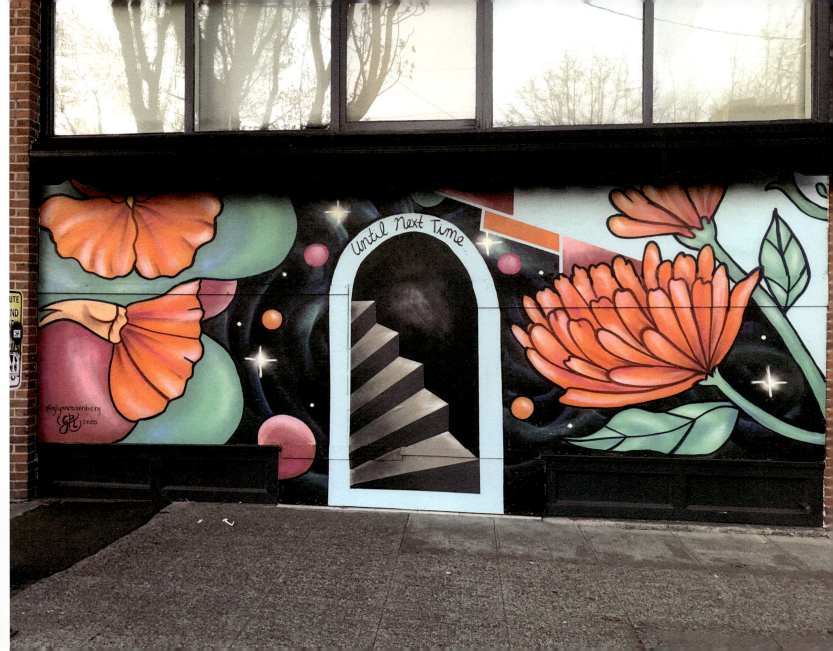

Artist: Haarald Peterson, Andi Imes
Crew: Taylor Reed
Name of Mural: *ALLONE*
Materials: 3/4" plywood, paint
Size: 8 x 12 feet
Location: Vacant Storefront, 2246 NW Market St
Coordinated by: Devin Reynolds
Artist's website: mach2arts.com

"I had surreptitiously placed the rhinoceros cutout as a guerrilla installation and then I added the gorilla. Just after that, Taylor Reed contacted me about a collaboration for that wall. Andi Imes, my neighbor, showed me a painting they had done and I thought it would go perfect in the blank space on that wall. We let the whole thing move organically. It wasn't as planned as some of the other murals that are so lovely, but it was a great experience that happened on its own."

—Haarald Peterson

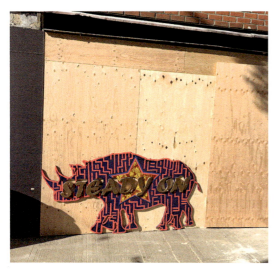

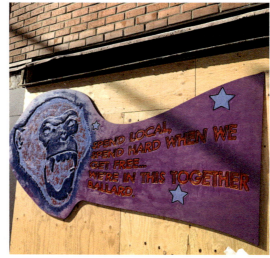

176   Photos: HAL PETERSON

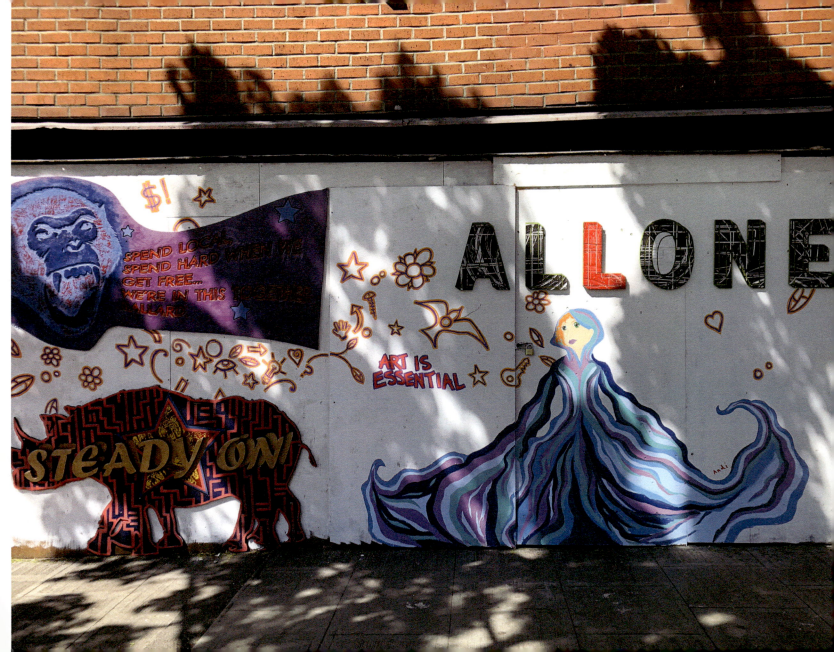

Artist:	Maryam Rouhfar
Crew:	Jeff Regelein
Name of Mural:	*Lookin' Out*
Materials:	Acrylic
Size:	5 x 10 feet
Location:	Old Volterra location on Ballard Ave
Coordinated by:	Bill and Ted's Excellent Adventures
Artist's website:	@m_a_r_o_u_h and @marrouhfar on Instagram

"I created Lookin' Out *as a symbol that we as a community and society are for the first time looking from the inside out. We are rediscovering ourselves in the midst of the chaos and reevaluating what is important, what we love, and how we can be excellent to each other."*

—Maryam Rouhfar

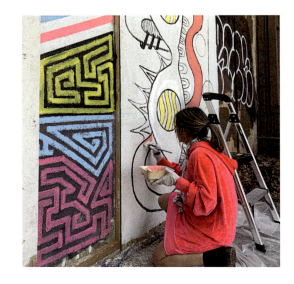
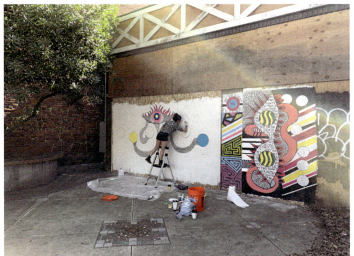

Photos: JEFF REGELEIN

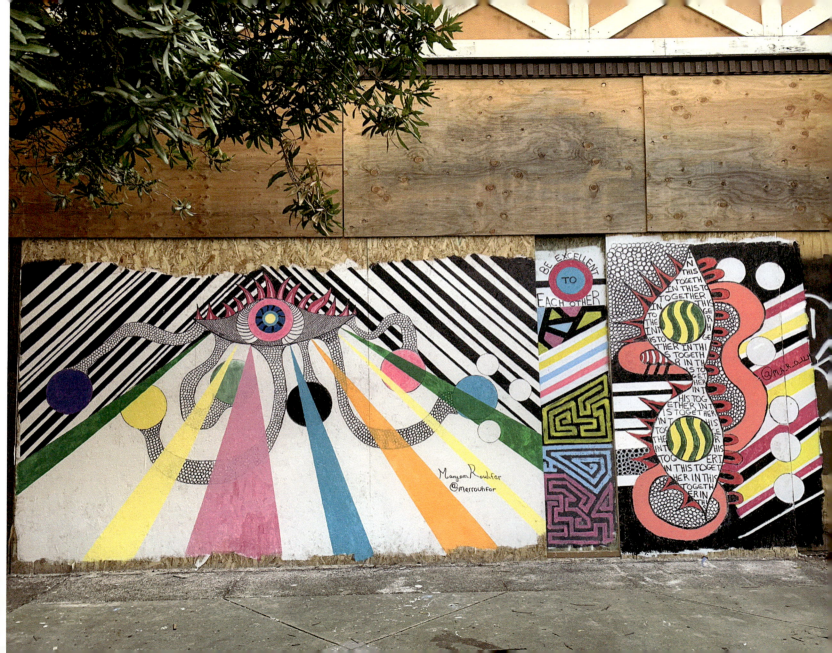

Artists:	Maryam Rouhfar
Name of Mural:	*BE.*
Materials:	Acrylic paint
Size:	3.5 x 3.5 feet
Location:	Kathy Casey Food Studios, 5130 Ballard Ave
Artist's website:	@marrouhfar on Instagram

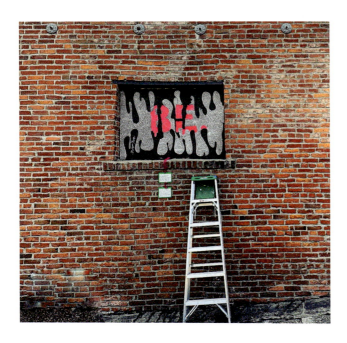

"This is meant as a message to all people that just being in this time of hardship and uncertainty is enough. It is a message to take the time to be thankful for existing in one of the hardest years of the 21st century."

—Maryam Rouhfar

180   **Photos:** AVA MOSTOFI

Artists:	Maryam Rouhfar
Name of Mural:	*The Yin to My Yang*
Materials:	Acrylic
Size:	4 x 10 feet
Location:	Bitterroot BBQ, 5239 Ballard Ave
Credits:	The Beatles
Artist's website:	@marrouhfar on Instagram

"I painted The Yin to My Yang *as a reminder that in order to see the light, we have to endure the darkness. This pandemic is allowing us the time and space to do so and to let things be as we grow and learn from what we don't have the luxury to experience anymore."*

—Maryam Rouhfar

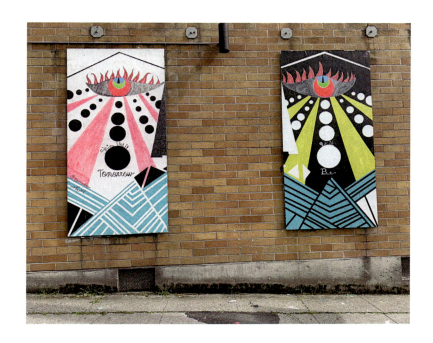

Photos: ARTIST

Artist:	Tori Shao
Crew:	Joshua Gawne
Name of Mural:	*Keep Calm Carry On, Keep Going Keep Growing*
Materials:	Exterior latex paint
Size:	6.5 x 22 feet
Location:	a&bé Bridal Shop Seattle, 5423 Ballard Ave NW
Coordinated by:	Devin Reynolds, Kiana Ballo
Artist's website:	torishao.com

"Growing up in Seattle, I have watched the Ballard neighborhood change and grow. When familiar and beloved businesses boarded up windows with plywood, the streets quickly transformed into disparaging scenes. These murals have helped to brighten up the streetscape during an uncertain time."

—Tori Shao

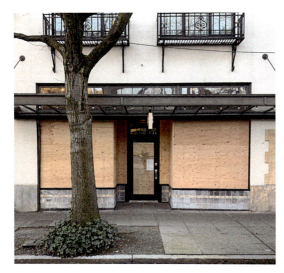
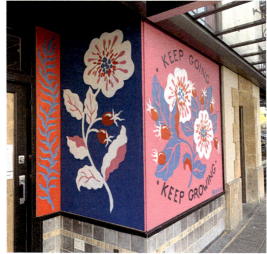

Photos: ARTISTS, DEVIN REYNOLDS

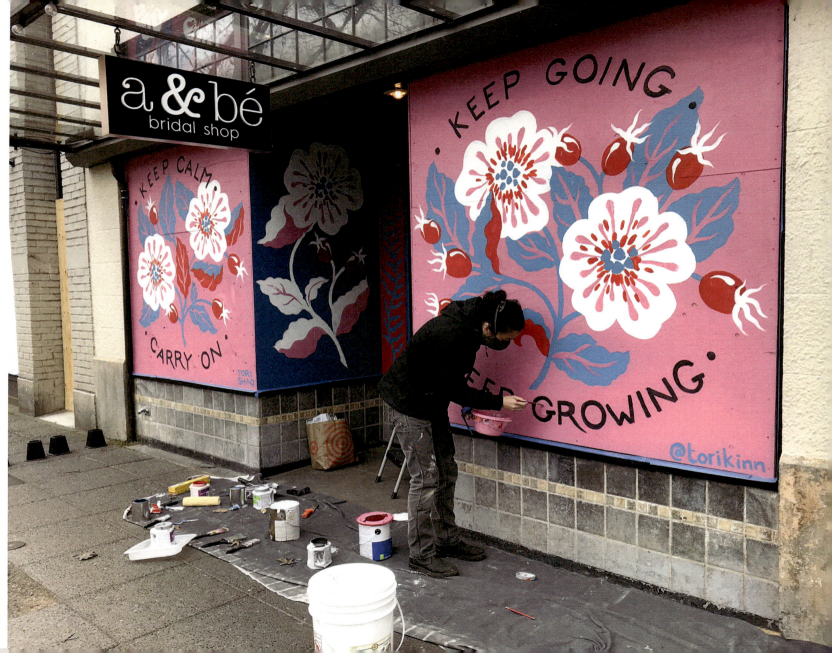

Artist: Tori Shao
Crew: Joshua Gawne
Name of Mural: *The Future is Bright*
Materials: Exterior latex paint
Size: 8.75 x 12.5 feet
Location: Ascent Outdoors, 5209 Ballard Ave NW
Coordinated by: Ballard Alliance: Devin Reynolds and Kiana Ballo
Artist's website: torishao.com

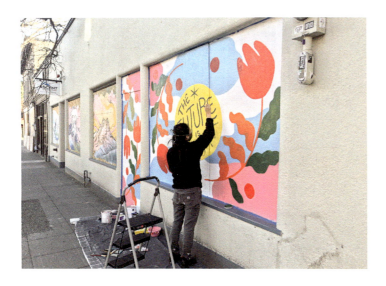

Photos: ARTISTS

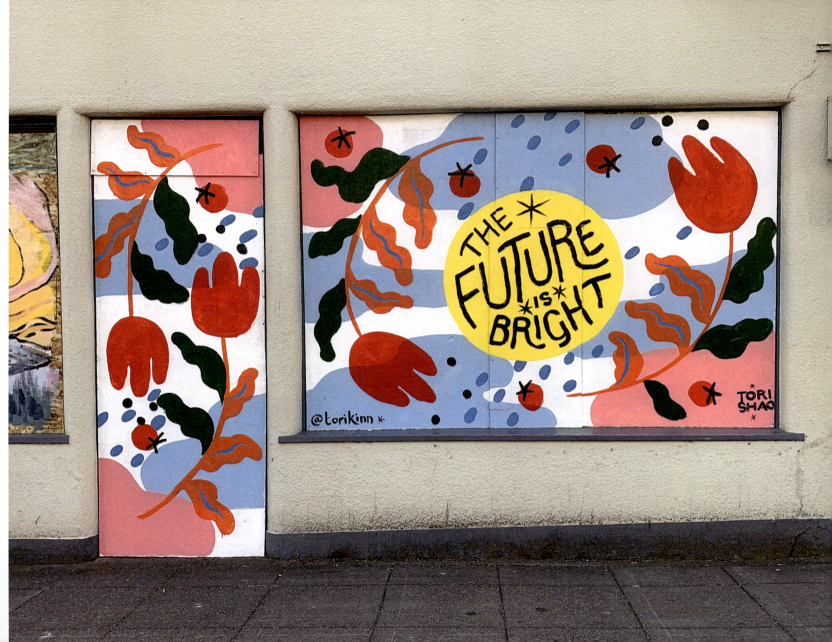

Artist: Tori Shao
Crew: Joshua Gawne
Name of Mural: *This Too Shall Pass*
Materials: Exterior latex paint
Size: 7 x 26.5 feet
Location: Horseshoe, 5344 Ballard Ave NW
Coordinated by: Devin Reynolds, Kiana Ballo
Artist's website: torishao.com

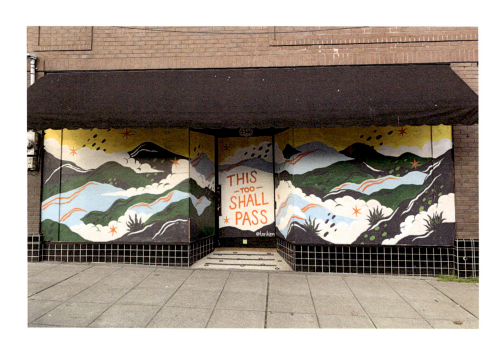

Photos: ARTISTS

Artists: Sean Mullin
Name of Mural: *Origami 1*
Materials: Paint
Size: 10 x 20 feet
Location: Kathy Casey Food Studios, 5130 Ballard Ave NW
Credits: Devin Reynolds, Ballard Alliance
Artist's website: @saint.jermain on Instagram

"Seattle has had a tenuous relationship with public art since I have lived in the city, but the plywood panels over storefronts have enabled a public art renaissance. I wish I had made it more explicitly political in nature, as was the initial intent, so as to emphasize how the "stay home, stay safe" discourse during the COVID-19 crisis is exclusionary to our unhoused friends and neighbors."

—Sean Mullin

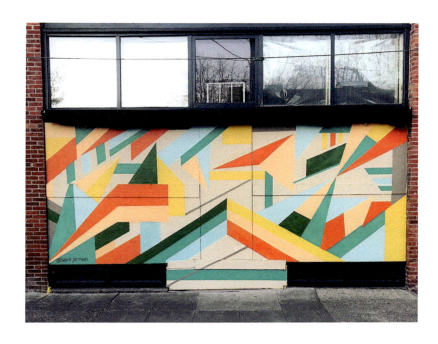

Photos: ARTIST

Wallingford
Greenwood

Artists: Jillian Chong
Name of Mural: *Surfin' Turtle*
Materials: Acrylic paint, spray paint, paint markers
Size: 8 x 4 feet
Location: Urban Surf, 2100 N Northlake Way
Artist's website: jillianchong.com

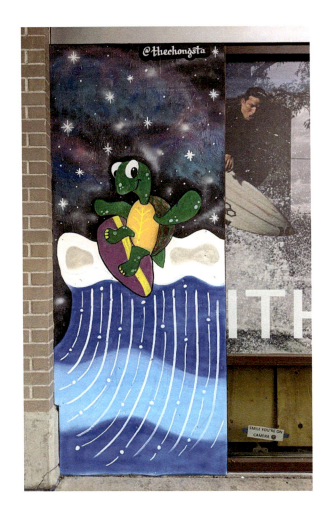

Photos: ARTIST

Artists: Robyn Emlen
Name of Mural: *True Wuv*
Materials: Spray paint
Size: 4 x 8 feet
Location: 4006 Wallingford Ave N
Artist's website: Inkbyrobyn.com

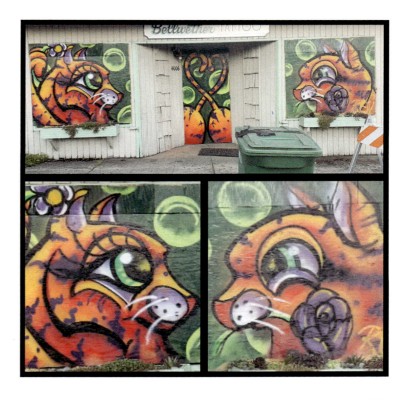

Photos: ARTIST

Artist:	Andrew Miller
Name of Mural:	*Party at Tim's Tavern*
Materials:	Acrylic house paint
Size:	8 x 28 feet
Location:	Tim's Tavern, 602 N 105th St
Coordinated by:	Mason Reed, owner
Artist's website:	mantisart.com

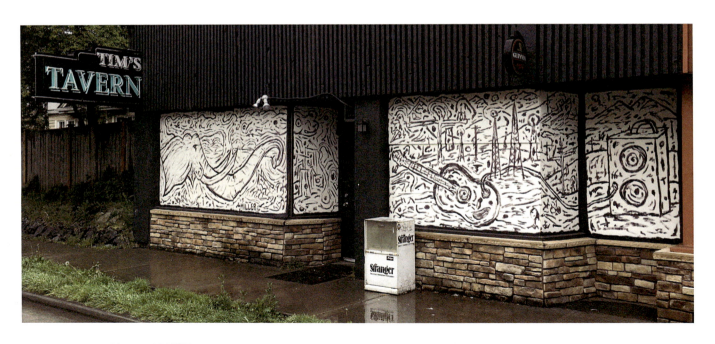

Photos: ARTIST

Artist: Andrew Miller
Name of Mural: *A1 Hummmmbird*
Materials: Acrylic house paint
Size: 8 x 12 feet
Location: A1 Hop Shop, 14401 Greenwood Ave N
Artist's website: mantisart.com

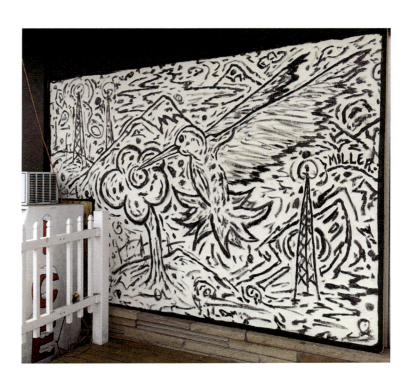

Photos: ARTIST

Georgetown
White Center

Artist: Sarah Robbins
Name of Mural: *Stay Safe White Center*
Materials: Latex paint
Size: 8 x 16 feet
Location: Beer Star and Lil Woodys, 9801 16th Ave SW
Artist's website: sarah-robbins.com

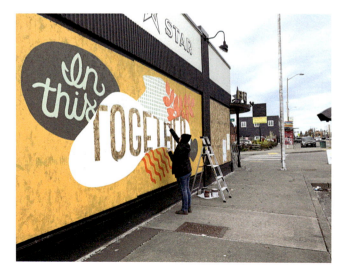 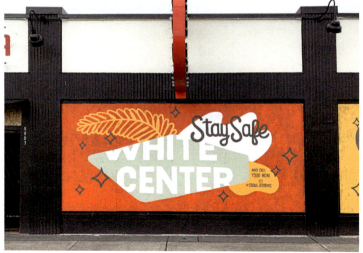

Photos: ARTIST

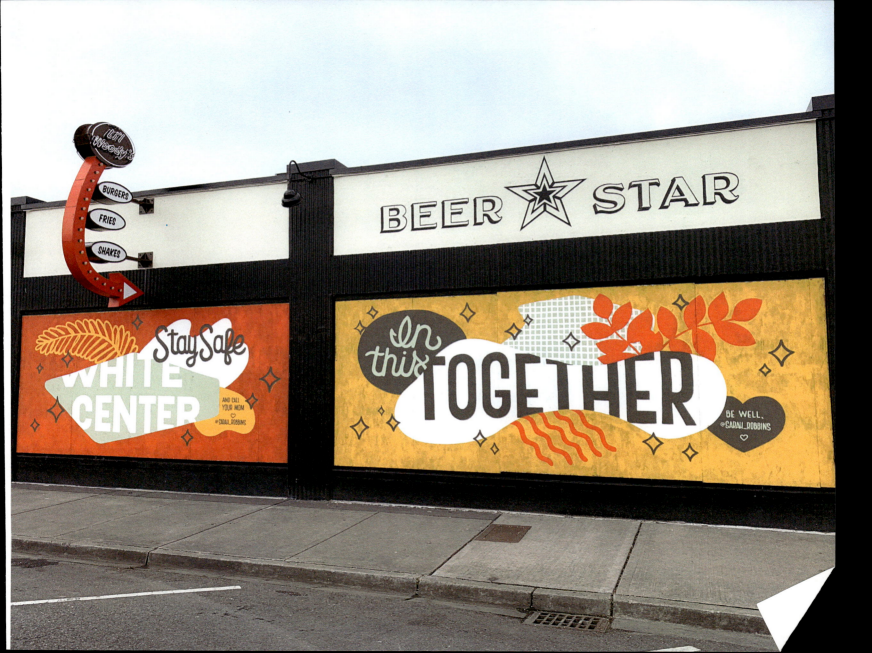

Artist: David Johansson
Name of Mural: *Call Your Mother, Happy Mothers Day 2020 Safety First*
Materials: Acrylic on plywood, Miller latex paint
Size: 8 x 18 feet
Location: District Vintage Home, 5531 Airport Way S
Artist's website: facebook.com/DavidJohanssonSeattle

"Call your mother. Every human mother deserves love and respect. For those of you who lost someone dear in 2020, may you find peace."

—David Johansson

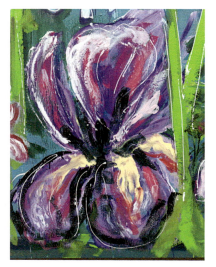
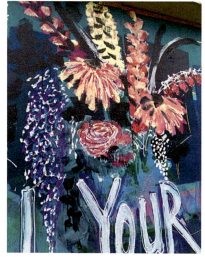
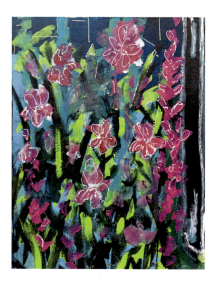

Photos: ARTIST

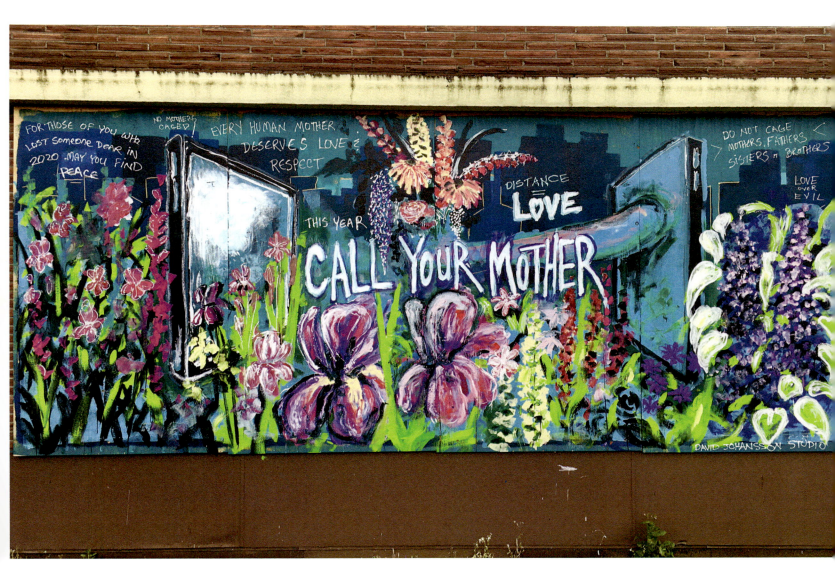

Artist:	David Johansson
Crew:	Simon Andrew Makhuli
Name of Mural:	*The Golden City Will Wait*
Materials:	Acrylic paint, 24 karat gold polymer
Size:	8 x 18 feet
Location:	Vacant Storefront, 6014 12th Ave S
Coordinated by:	Patti Curtis Fogue Gallery
Artist's website:	facebook.com/DavidJohanssonSeattle

"*The Golden City Will Wait* depicts trees running towards the city, with multiple space needles throughout. The needles represent hope, and the 24k gold paint represents the economic success that Seattle is known for. The magic of this painting is reminiscent of the fabled Emerald City."

—David Johansson

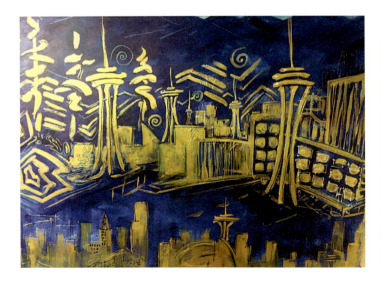

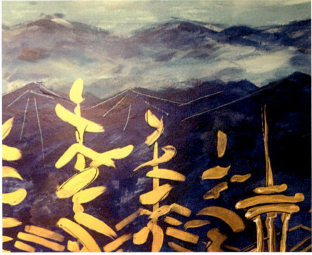

Photos: ARTIST

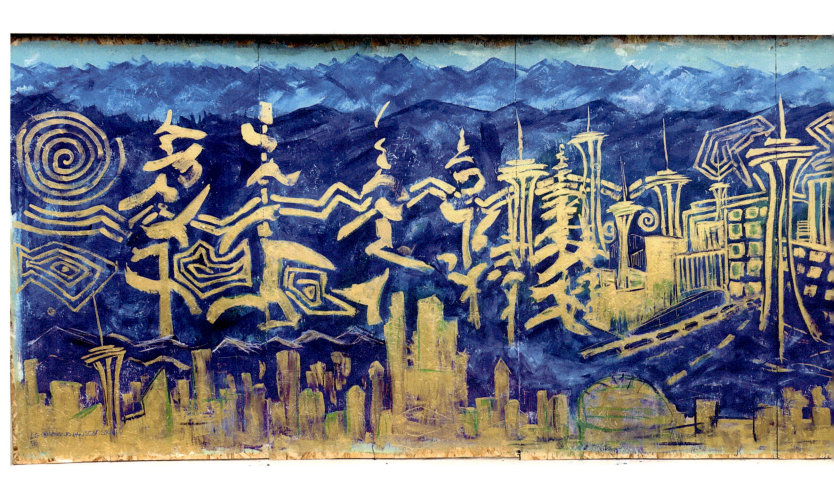

Artists:	David Johansson
Crew:	Simon Andrew Makhuli
Name of Mural:	*Washington Grateful*
Materials:	Acylic paint
Size:	12 x 16 feet
Location:	District Vintage, 5531 Airport Way S
Coordinated by:	Patti Curtis
Artist's website:	facebook.com/DavidJohanssonSeattle

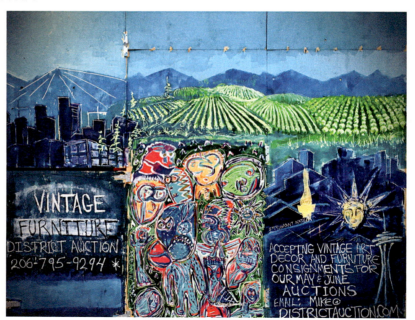

Photos: ARTIST

Artists:	David Johansson
Name of Mural:	*The Mountain Watches*
Materials:	Acrylic paint
Size:	8 x 8 feet
Location:	Artcore Tattoo Studios, 5501 Airport Way S
Coordinated by:	John Bennett
Artist's website:	facebook.com/DavidJohanssonSeattle

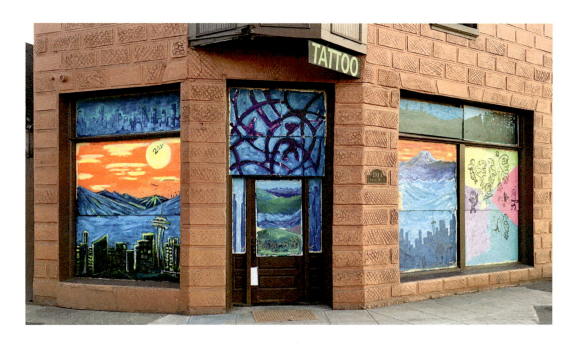

Photos: ARTIST

Artists:	David Johansson
Crew:	Simon Andrew Makhuli
Name of Mural:	*New York Calm Before the Storm*
Materials:	Acrylic paint
Size:	8 x 18 feet
Location:	District Vintage, 5531 Airport Way S
Coordinated by:	Patti Curtis
Artist's website:	facebook.com/DavidJohanssonSeattle

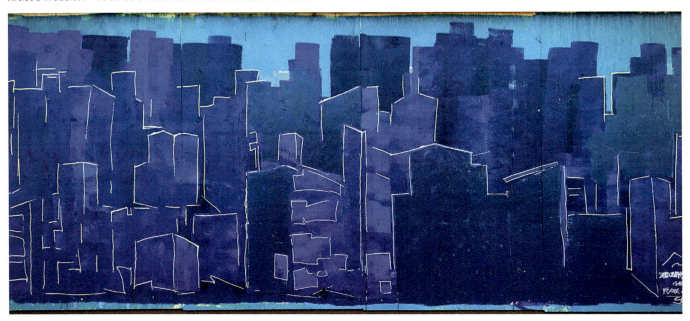

Photos: ARTIST

Columbia City

Artist: Jake Millett
Name of Mural: *Weather the Storm*
Materials: House paint, spray paint, paint pen
Size: 5 x 3 feet each
Location: Lottie's Lounge, 4900 Rainier Ave S
Artist's website: jakemillett.com

"I felt compelled to add a little art, color, and love to my neighborhood as we cope with the pandemic together."

—Jake Millett

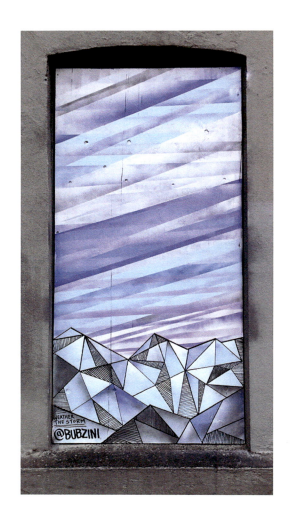

Photos: ARTIST

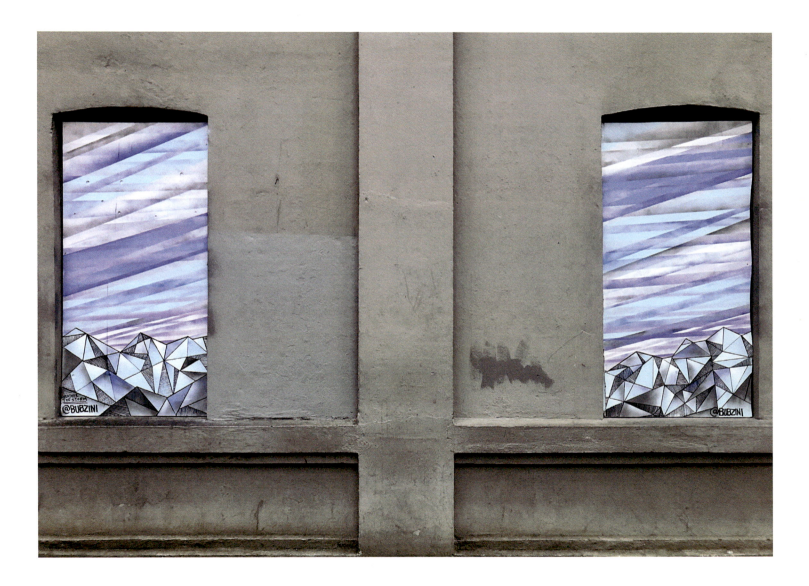

Artist: Burgandy Viscosi
Name of Mural: *Healthy Lungs*
Materials: Acrylic paint
Size: 6 x 10 feet
Location: CrossFit, 4243 Rainier Ave S
Artist's website: burgandyviscosi.com

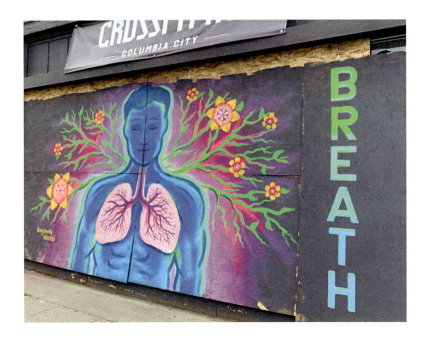

Photos: MATTHEW MACDONALD

Artist: Sandy
Name of Mural: *Cats of the Day*
Materials: Rustoleum on latex
Size: 6 x 7 feet
Location: Molly Moon's, 4822 Rainier Ave S
Artist's website: @paint_2_change on Instagram

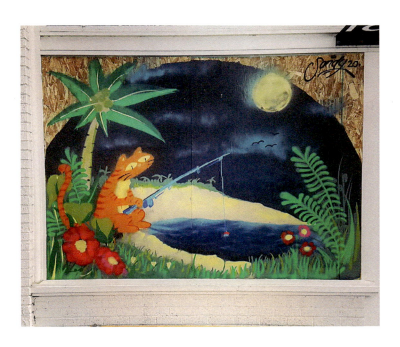

Photos: MATTHEW MACDONALD

Acknowledgements and Thanks

We would like to thank all the people who helped make this book possible, including:

Amanda Joyce Bishop, Ty Kreft & the amazing Dot for making the Arundel Books mural possible. Kathleen Warren and the folks at Overall Creative, for your help with that, and for your work connecting so many people in so many ways. Neil Gaiman, Merrilee Heifetz & the great folks at Writers House, for letting us publish the *A Book is a Dream* mural as a poster, and starting us thinking about turning the storefront murals into a book.

Sara Pizzo of the Alliance for Pioneer Square, Seth Geiser at the DSA, Devin Reynolds of the Ballard Alliance, Katy Ricchiuto at the U-District Partnership, Lauren Ross at the SODO BIA, for your help connecting us with artists.

Ian Crozier, for your capable enthusiasm and saying yes to co-creating a whole map in one day, showcasing the sites of murals as they were going up all over the city, and for being willing to update it with dozens more sites just a month or so later. Your love for vibrant urban spaces is contagious.

Jean Sherrard, of the *Seattle Times* "Now & Then" feature, Margo Vansynghel and Brangien Davis of Crosscut.org, Deborah Horne, KIRO 7 television, the folks at Shelf Awareness, the team at *The Stranger*, and the other folks in the media who so kindly helped get the word out.

Our fabulous summer intern Malia Maxwell, for wrangling a whole lot of data points, and generally making a big, short-deadline project feel manageable. To Cyra Jane Hobson for your amazing work with images, layout, and text. To Jessica Levey for your skills and enthusiasm, and Joanne Aquino for helping spread awareness. And to Dean Kelly, for running all over the city, reaching out to help connect us with artists, and helping inspire us to really *do* this book.

And most of all thanks to the artists, for putting your faith in our team to create something worthy of your amazing work, and for your courage in a dark time to bring light to the people of this city.

Viva Seattle!

—Phil Bevis and Annie Brulé, co-publishers,
ChatwinBooks

Viral Creativity: COVID-19 Murals on Seattle Storefronts

GREENWOOD

BALLARD

FREMONT

QUEEN ANNE

CAPITOL HILL

DOWNTOWN

BELLTOWN

PIONEER SQUARE

CHINATOWN/ID

SODO

COLUMBIA CITY

GEORGETOWN

IN SPRING 2020, AS THE COVID-19 pandemic forced hundreds of businesses to close their doors and board their windows, the role of main streets in Seattle transformed. Artists, community leaders, businesses, and funders sprang into action to create vibrant, wildly diverse, uplifting art on boarded-up storefronts to inspire generosity, patience, and solidarity during difficult times. The transformation of main streets into public galleries within a few weeks reminds us how **vibrant community places help to build resilience**, and of the wealth of latent creativity we posses, just looking for a canvas.

*We know there to be many more murals than the 100+ we currently have documentation for, and more are appearing each day...

MAP BY Annie Brulé (Vashon Island, Washington, USA: 47.396370, -122.465570) and Ian Crozier (Seattle, Washington, USA 47.6212638, -122.3202837). All murals created in March, April, and May 2020. **THIS DATA** was collected from the artists by Annie's publishing company, Chatwin Books, which is currently publishing a book on Seattle's COVID-19 murals, due out in mid 2020. **MURALS PICTURED** are by: (from top left) Shogo Ota, Cady Bogart, Leo Shallat, Sara Pizzo, C.M. Ruiz, Baso Fibonacci, Sean Mullin, (from bottom left) ZachRockstad, Dozfy the Artist, David Johansson Studio, @TheyDrift and @ksra_ksra, Hal Peterson, Chris Kent, Eos Montana, and (inset) Reed Olsen. **MAP CREATED ON** 05.15.2020 for *Atlas in a Day #2: Community*, by Guerrilla Cartography.

Donors and Sponsors

with our thanks

Anonymous: who made twenty copies of this book free to the mural artists

Jamie Merriman-Cohen

Katherine Reynolds

Arundel Books

Brulé Illustration & Design

Index

8oz Burger & Co—118
a&bé Bridal Shop—182-183
A1 Hop Shop—193
Adana—83, 98, 109, 120
Agate Designs—44-45
Allen, Kelsey—70
Alliance for Pioneer Square—14-15, 18-19,
        24-25, 27, 31, 34
Altstadt Bierhalle & Brathaus—35
Alyea, Rosie—74
Alyn, Nicole—54, 66-67
Amber Seattle—65, 69
Angelou, Maya—92
Art Primo—151, 168
Artcore Tattoo Studios—203
ArtXchange Gallery—32-33
Arundel Books—10-11
Ascent Outdoors—184-185
Atire—99
Atwood, Margaret—24
Avery, Billie—62
AxeHAKA—78-79
B Line Dot—12-13
Ballard Alliance—163-167, 184-185, 187
Ballard Annex—165
Ballo, Kiana—182-186
The Baltic Room—101
Barbre, Crystal—20, 82, 84-85
Barely Awake—100-102
The Beatles—181
Beer Star—196-197
Belltown Pizza—63, 68, 71-72

Bennett, Dillon—56
Bennett, John—203
Big Mario's—151
Bill and Ted's Excellent Adventures
        —178-179
Bishop, Amanda Joyce—10-11, 74
Bitteroot BBQ—181
Bogart, Cady—81
Bon Voyage Vintage—18-19
Broadway Market Complex—88
Buttnick Building—38-39, 46
C. M. Ruiz—80
Café Campagne—52-53
Cantwell, Jessica—59-60
Capitol Cider—97
Capitol Coffee Works—117
Carlino, Nick—160
Carlino, Trish—160
Castle Megastore—92, 102, 113
The Central Saloon—47
CES Studio—128-129
Chase Bank—116
Cho, Caroline—55
Choinere, Kalee Bly—see Barely Awake
Cholewinksi, Lina—70, 103, 143
Chong, Jillian—94-96, 136-137, 190
Chu Minh—141
Cinnaholic—95, 97
City Hostel—63
Comet Tavern—74, 81
Conor Byrne Pub—164
Conover, Katie—121

Copymart—136-137
Corn, Sallyann—21
Counter Culture Coffee—14-15
Counterbalance Barber Shop—152
CrossFit—208
Curtis, Patti—200-201, 204
Day, Sam—42-43
Dean, Christina—59-60
Delmar Building—31
Derschang, Linda—72, 172
Devil's Triangle—51
Dickinson, Ezra—89
District—198-199, 202, 204
The Doctor's Office—134
Doghouse Leathers—104-105
Downtown Seattle Association—59-60
Downtown Seattle Cares—50
Dozfy, LLC—see Dozfy
Dozfy—54, 55, 64-69, 83, 134, 153, 169-172
Drake, Kevin—90-91
Efflux Creations—see Lobuzzetta, Lance
Ego—18-19
Eido—22-23
Emerald City Guitars—34
Emlen, Robyn—191
Esters Enoteca—160
Evans, Conor—12-13
Feely, Brandon—12-13
Fern the cat—71
Fibonacci, Baso—14-15
Files, Patrick—164
Fillingim, Sharon—153

Fischer, Jonathan Wakuda—32-33, 36-67
Fitzgerald, Joanna—58
Flatstick Pub—27-29
Fogue Gallery—200-201
fruitsuper SHOP—21
Gaiman, Neil—10-11
Gallery Erato—20
Gawne, Joshua—182-186
Geiser, Seth—50
George and Dragon—158
Globe Bookstore—42-43
Gnartoons—25
Goldsuit—90-91
Good Bar—26, 30
Gorder, Hanna—93
The Grand Central Building—25
Gray Sky Gallery—12-13
Guido—99
Hale, Devon Midori—52-53
Halladay, Alex—18-19
Hawks Nest—144-146
Heartwood Provisions—66-67
Hiatt, Bailee—118, 159
Holloway, Dawna—21
Honor Coffee—130-131
Horseshoe—186
Hubner, Katlyn—104-105
Hunnicutt, Beverly—150
Imes, Andi—176-177
J&M Café—48
Jackson, Michael—89
James the Stanton—see Gnartoons
Jerrett, Michael—65, 68
Johansson, David—198-204
Josephon-Day, Anna—93

Jujubeet—22-23
Kathy Casey Food Studio—166, 174-175, 180, 187
Kent, Joe—21
KEXP—89
Kinesia Pilates Studio—24
King's Hardware—172
Kovalik, Vladimir—34, 47, 93
Kreau—130-134
Kreft, Ty—10-11
Ksra—122-123
Kubota Gardens—109
Laughing Buddha Tattoo—112
Le Labo—106-107
Lee Properties—150, 165
Lee, Brian—55, 71-72
Lennon, John—71
Life on Mars—76-77, 84-85, 89, 126-127
Lil Woody's—196-197
LillyBomb—144-145
Linda Derschang Group—128-129
Linda's Tavern—80, 129
Lobuzzetta, Lance—31
Lost Lake Cafe—75, 90-91
Lottie's Lounge—206-207
Love, Jada—22-23
Lucca's Great Finds—170-171
Luna, Claudia Castro—40-41
Maes, Shavonee—71
Main—99
Maione, Michael—55
Makhuli, Simon Andrew—200-202, 204
Malover, Bekah—166-167
The Market Arms—162
Martin, Mackenzie—12-13

Mason, Jay—27-29
Massagli, Camillo—76-77
McDonald's—59-60
Mean Sandwich—169
Metropolitan Grill—54
Michael Lee—see Lee Properties
Midgley, Matt—108
Miller, Andrew—148-150, 162-165, 192-193
Millett, Jake—92-93, 206-207
Molly Moon's—209
Monde, Ray—40-41
Montgomery, Mason—35
Morgan—117
Mosef—99
Mullin, Sean—187
Nakajima, Shota—98, 120
National Corporate Housing—142
Neumos—119
Nieri, Dom—26, 30
Nix, Joe—30
Nordstrom—57
Novo Painting—167
Nunn, Paul—38-39
Oddfellows—96
Olafssen, Phineas—22-23
Old Navy—58
Oliveira, Sophia—58
Olsen, Reed—146
Oostra, Erin—24
Ota, Shogo—1120
Overall Creative—10-11, 35, 48, 62, 70, 74-75, 81, 84-85, 88-89, 93, 100, 103, 106-108, 112-116, 124-129, 144-146
Palihotel—50
Parrow, Ariel—50, 75, 142

Patagonia—168
Pertl, Miles—44-45
Pertl, Sydney M.—44-45
Peterson, Haarald—176-177
Petrovic, Tija—22-23
Pioneer Smoke—14-15
Pizzo, Sara—20, 22-23, 27-29, 40-41, 44-45
Pizzuto, Mia—109
Pohl, Sara—97
Prestes, Sabrina—58
Prine, John—126-127
Proulx, Gretchen—136-137
QFC—99
Queen City—63, 72
Quinn's Pub—94, 102, 132-133
Re-Bar—51
Reed, Mason—192
Reed, Taylor—176-177
Regelein, Jeff—178-179
Rejuvenation—143
Retail Therapy—86
Reynolds, Devin—151, 166-171, 174-177, 182-187
Rice, Josephine—96-98, 173
Richards, John—89
Rilke, Rainer Maria—76-77
Ritual—78-79
Rivelle, Ethan—87
Robbins, Sarah—59-60, 196-197
Rockstad, Zach—126-127
Roq La Rue—82
Rosenberg, Glynn—174-175
Ross, Lauren—56, 142-143
Rouhfar, Maryam—178-181

Ruby—99
Rudy's Barbershop—62, 159, 167, 169
The Runaway—124-125, 128
Saeteun's Garage—see Saeteun
Saeteun—140
Saint John's—134
Salsa Con Todo—156-157
Sam's Tavern—95, 110-111
Sandy—57, 69, 99, 116-119, 140, 156-159, 209
Schlough, Will—124-125
Seahorse Bar—63
SeaPertl Productions—44-45
Sexton, Karl—64
Shallat, Leo—34, 47
Shao, Tori—182-186
Shibuya, Mari—36-37, 106-107
Shingletown Saloon—172
Showgirls—51
Siems, Anne—76-77
Siscoe, Joe—42-43
Sloop Tavern—164
Sneaker City—55
Some Random Bar—55, 71
Spillman, Sam—12-13
St. Charles, Genevieve—90-91
Stedman, Joel—148-149
Stevens, Rich M.—113
Stitches—96
Strathern, Evann—88, 103
STT Lettering—56
Sugar, Rebecca—112
Swannie's Sports Bar—40-41
SYCO—99
Takasawa, Zach—84-85

Tardiff, Rob—70
Targy's Tavern—148-149
Tashiro Kaplan Artists Loft—16-17
Tay, Rainbow—112
Taylor, Ronnie—114-115
Terada, Leah—44-45
They Drift—122-123
Tieu, Kimberly—62, 103
Tim's Tavern—192
Tonnu, Marry—126-127
Tractor Tavern—163
Trout, Sam—103
Urban Artworks—57
Urban Outfitters—93, 100, 103, 108
Urban Surf—190
Varchetta, Antonio—141, 151, 168
Velan, Tara—46, 71-72, 119, 121, 160
Venue Ballard—173
The Virginia Inn—64
Viscosi, Burgandy—51, 63, 86, 152, 208
Visit Ballard—174-175
VK Signs—106-107
Volterra—178-179
Vue Lounge—70
Warren, Kathleen—75-77, 81, 89-91, 97, 103, 114-115, 144-145
Washington Nightlife Music Association —119
Weldon, Casey—18-19, 82, 84-85
Whitehead, Sam—87
Wildrose—87, 121
Williams, Carol Rashawnna—16-17
Witte, Japhy—26, 96, 98
Zaeos—48, 128-129
Zion, Moran—110-111